5/04

ConsumerLab.com's

GUIDE TO
Buying
Vitamins &
Supplements

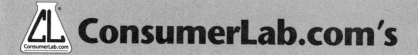

ConsumerLab.com's

GUIDE TO

Buying
Vitamins &
Supplements

What's _really_ in the bottle?

Edited by Tod Cooperman, M.D.,
William Obermeyer, Ph.D., and
Densie Webb, R.D., Ph.D.

ConsumerLab.com, LLC, White Plains, New York 10605
© 2003 by ConsumerLab.com All rights reserved

11 10 09 08 07 06 05 04 03   10 9 8 7 6 5 4 3

Printed in Canada

Library of Congress Cataloging-in-Publication Data

ConsumerLab.com's guide to buying vitamins & supplements : what's really in the bottle? / by the Staff of ConsumerLab.com ; edited by Tod Cooperman, William Obermeyer, and Denise Webb.
  p. ; cm.
Includes index.
ISBN 0-9729697-0-5 (pbk. : alk. paper)
1. Dietary supplements—Popular works. 2. Vitamins—Popular works.
3. Consumer education.
[DNLM: 1. Vitamins—standards. 2. Dietary Supplements—standards.
3. Plant Preparations—standards. 4. Product Surveillance,
Postmarketing. QU 160 C758 2003] I. Title: Guide to buying vitamins & supplements. II. Cooperman, Tod. III. Obermeyer, William. IV. Webb, Densie, R.D. V. ConsumerLab.com, LLC. V. Title.
RM258.5.C66 2003
613.2'8—dc21
2003005665

To all who have wondered
what is really in the bottle.

CONTENTS

PART 3
PRODUCT REVIEWS FOR
HERBALS AND OTHER SUPPLEMENTS

APPENDICES

TABLES

PREFACE

S
ince 1999 ConsumerLab.com has independently tested dietary supplements and reported the results online at www.consumerlab.com. Hundreds of thousands of people have come to the site to essentially "look under the hood" of these products to find out whether or not what is inside the bottle is the same as the label's claim. Many readers have written to tell us how sorely needed this information is and how the information has directed them toward more effective and safer products.

We have also heard from people asking us to make this information accessible without a computer. With the publication of this book, we are pleased to provide 3 years of our research and information to readers and to present the material in a format that's convenient to access on a regular basis. We hope this information, too, will be helpful.

In addition, we hope a more educated and discerning public will inevitably lead to further improvements in product quality, as manufacturers strive to meet consumers' demands.

The information in this book is based on our knowledge in 2002. Because testing continues and new information about supplements is always coming out, I encourage you to stay up-to-date by joining our free E-mail list and subscribing to our online information at www.consumerlab.com.

Tod Cooperman, M.D.
President and Founder
ConsumerLab.com

Acknowledgments

The editors wish to express their appreciation to Lisa Sabin, Vice President of Business Development at ConsumerLab.com, for her assistance at every step. We also thank our families: whenever a difficult decision had to be made, we thought of you and the answer became clear.

INTRODUCTION

How to use this guide

If you've ever wondered what's in a supplement—say vitamin C, calcium, fish oil, or ginseng—then you've joined scores of consumers with similar questions. You wonder whether to pay extra for vitamin C with rose hips. Then, there's the calcium dilemma: Some calcium products, reports indicate, are better absorbed than others and some products don't dissolve well. But which is which? As for fish oils, labeled dosages vary considerably. What's the recommended dosage for your condition? And ginseng? Does the plant species matter? Most important: Do the products—which no government agency routinely checks for quality—contain the ingredients claimed on their labels?

Wonder no more. ConsumerLab.com's Guide to Buying Vitamins & Supplements: What's Really in the Bottle? has the answers to those questions and dozens like them. This consumer-friendly volume—the first of its kind on supplements—packs a no-nonsense look at supplements, but no hype.

To get the most from ConsumerLab.com's Guide to Buying Vitamins & Supplements, peruse "Part 1: Why test?" first. It provides valuable background about the government's role in monitoring and regulating supplement production and labeling. Chapter 2, also in part 1, gives an overview of nine problems you can encounter with supplements. These problems range from none or little of the claimed ingredient in the product—a concern most commonly associated with expensive supplements such as chondroitin and SAMe—to poor disintegration—typically a concern with calcium and multivitamins. There's more: In "Herbal alert," you'll find a detailed discussion of 11 herbs that are best avoided. This short chapter is recommended reading if you're inclined to use herbal supplements.

"Part 2: Product reviews for vitamins and minerals" and "Part 3 Product reviews for herbal and other supplements" account for more than half of ConsumerLab.com's Guide to Buying Vitamins & Supplements and provide a close look at products tested by ConsumerLab.com. It, along with other independent laboratories, evaluated more than 350 supplement brands. Careful reading of these sections will supply the necessary information for making consumer-smart supplement choices. Each product review includes this information: main ingredient description, test findings, quality brands, recommended dosage, consumer tips, and more.

To read about new recalls, warnings, and evaluations, visit the ConsumerLab.com web site, www.consumerlab.com.

PART ONE

Why test?

CHAPTER 1

Buyer beware

When we started ConsumerLab.com in 1999, consumers had no way of knowing what their dietary supplements contained. At the time, scattered reports suggested that supplements might not live up to their claims, but no comprehensive source of information was available.

To remedy the information shortfall and determine whether products met their claims, we purchased and tested, over a three-year time span, hundreds of supplements, including vitamins, minerals, herbals, creatine, fish oils, glucosamine, SAMe, and MSM. The results were shocking: About one-quarter of the products didn't pass the evaluations.

Some categories of supplements fared better than others. For example, of the B vitamins tested only 5% had problems. In contrast, other products performed remarkably poorly. Specifically, 15% of the vitamins and minerals, 38% of the herbals, and 23% of the other supplements failed our testing. Some individual products, such as the herbal ginseng, performed even worse: 59% of the products tested had problems.

The 20 categories of products covered in this book make up the vast majority of supplements sold in the United States. ConsumerLab.com evaluated more than 500 products representing 157 different brands. The products failing our evaluations came from every type and size of company. In addition, where the products were purchased—pharmacy, health food store, catalog, or other outlet—had no bearing on whether they passed the tests. No channel of distribution was immune to failure.

Why products fail

Supplements didn't pass our evaluations for many reasons. The most common problem we encountered was too little or none of the main ingredient. Other reasons included too much active ingredient, the wrong ingredient, dangerous or illegal ingredients, contamination (with heavy metals, dangerous pesticides, or pathogens), unexpected ingredients ("spiked" products), poor disintegration (which affects absorption), misleading or insufficient product information, and misleading or unsupported health claims. Each problem is discussed in detail in other sections of the book. (See "9 Common concerns," page 8, and individual product reviews.)

The role of regulators

In 2000, the estimated cost of developing a new prescription drug and getting it to the U.S. market was $329 million. A dietary supplement, however, can be produced and brought to market for just a few thousand dollars.

WHY THE DISPARITY?

Prescription drugs must be proven safe and effective and must be manufactured under rigorous conditions. In addition, drug packaging must indicate exactly what the product contains, and the contents can be no more than 10% over the labeled amount. The package must also provide extensive literature explaining the drug's approved uses, potential adverse effects, and the risks associated with the drug's use, including known interactions with foods or other drugs. Drug companies must meet all these requirements to the satisfaction of the U.S. Food and Drug Administration (FDA) before marketing a drug.

Dietary supplements, on the other hand, don't require proof that they work or that they're safe. Although supplement labels are supposed to state exactly what's in the package, no governmental agency routinely checks for compliance. And although supplements may make general, government-approved statements about ways in which they may help or maintain normal body functioning, neither manufacturers nor distributors are required to back the statements with research or provide information about the uses, adverse effects, or risks. Except for a few specific, preauthorized health claims, supplement labels aren't supposed to include claims about treating, diagnosing, or preventing disease — but some do anyway. Unlike prescription drugs, supplements aren't required to be manufactured under specific standardized conditions.

Once a prescription drug is on the market, the FDA monitors the drug's production and its performance for unforeseen adverse effects and interactions. Manufacturers and physicians must report adverse reactions to drugs, and systems for reporting, collecting, storing, and distributing such information are in place. If new evidence of a problem arises or if a manufacturing error occurs, drugs may be pulled from the market to ensure public safety.

It's rare, however, that the FDA recalls an unsafe supplement. The reason: no agency requires physicians or manufacturers to report adverse reactions and no strong, centralized system collects reports. Moreover, supplement manufacturers aren't required to maintain records of reported adverse reactions to their products, and no centralized system for reviewing data exists. The FDA does keep a database of adverse effects, but the database hasn't been updated since 1998. When the occasional recall occurs, the supplement company may quietly notify distributors and retailers, but it probably won't notify the public. The few recalls that are made public or are initiated by the FDA are reported on the FDA's web site. But even these recalls aren't always well communicated to the public. (Reported recalls can generally be found on ConsumerLab.com's web site under Recalls and Warnings — http://www.consumerlab.com/recalls.asp.)

In 1994, the government passed the Dietary Supplement Health and Education Act (commonly referred to as DSHEA or "de-shay"). This law doesn't classify dietary supplements as "drugs" and, therefore, has allowed them to fall outside the realm of FDA's regulation of prescription drugs. (In some other countries, most notably Germany, supplements are classified as drugs and are regulated as such.) U.S. law, however, does distinguish supplements from foods. Consequently, the Department of Agriculture (USDA), which regulates agricultural products including foods and beverages, doesn't regulate or oversee supplements. For example, though the USDA routinely inspects imported meat, no one routinely inspects imported supplements or their raw ingredients.

A 1998 amendment to the DSHEA has allowed manufacturers to make general claims, called "structure or function" claims about their products' benefits. Examples of such claims include "helps promote healthy skin," "helps improve strength and agility," and "helps improve cardiovascular fitness." Thanks to these claims, the marketing of supplements boomed, as did the market itself. Consumers rushed to buy the supplements, often attracted by their "natural" ingredients, rarely questioning product usefulness or quality. Sales of supplements increased from $2 billion in 1985 to $15 billion in 1995.

In the late 1990s, sales of supplements, particularly herbals, began to slow. Why? The reason isn't clear, but consumers may have read several of the published studies that didn't support the claimed benefits of certain supplements, such as ginseng. Or it's possible that people who purchased inferior products didn't buy more. Of all the supplements tested, ConsumerLab.com has found that herbals have the highest rate of failure.

Looking ahead

Both the government and supplement industry are taking steps to correct overstated claims and shortfalls in quality control. For starters, the National Institutes of Health (NIH) has initiated several major clinical studies to determine the effectiveness of some popular supplements, such as ginkgo biloba, saw palmetto, and valerian. Equally important, industry trade groups have begun to acknowledge that poor-quality products are a problem and that people won't buy products that don't work. Consequently, the industry has begun to call for good manufacturing practices (GMPs) on a voluntary and self-enforced basis.

The FDA is also moving toward requiring the use of GMPs. Such a ruling would call for a third party to ensure proper record keeping during manufacturing. However, the ruling won't become law and be implemented for several years. And unfortunately, the law won't have provisions for actively monitoring GMPs. Even at their best, GMPs can't fix all problems. Bad products could still be manufactured because the proposed GMPs will allow for a manufacturer's discretion as to product content, including either too much or too little of the key ingredient, untested combinations of ingredients, and poor quality of starting materials.

Nevertheless, improvements are slowly being made. For example, after ConsumerLab.com discovered problem products, some manufacturers upgraded manufacturing practices, secured more reliable ingredient suppliers, and corrected labeling deficiencies. But consumers should be aware that supplements commonly remain on shelves for two to three years, so newer products may be next to older ones on store shelves for years to come. Still, consumers must remember that prescription drugs receive stringent regulation and oversight compared to that of vitamins, minerals, herbals, and other supplements. Even over-the-counter drugs for coughs, colds, allergies, and hemorrhoids are scrutinized more than supplements. Buyer beware.

CHAPTER 2

9 Common concerns

W hat's really in the supplement bottle? If it isn't what you think, the supplement could be useless or, even worse, dangerous. What's also scary is that you can take a poor-quality supplement for an extended period without knowing there's a problem. For example, St. John's wort normally takes a few weeks before its antidepressant effect becomes apparent. So if you were to take the supplement for several weeks and not see an improvement, you wouldn't know whether the product lacks the active ingredient or it just isn't helping you. Another example: You take calcium to help prevent osteoporosis. But what if the supplement is deficient? Will you eventually develop osteoporosis? And if you do, will you know that too little calcium in your supplement may be the cause? Unfortunately, too little ingredient isn't the only supplement problem. Some products also have contaminants that can cause immediate or future health problems.

The following are the 9 most common problems ConsumerLab.com encountered during testing:

- Too little or no active ingredient
- Too much active ingredient
- Wrong ingredient
- Dangerous or illegal ingredients
- Contamination
- Unexpected ingredients ("spiked" products)
- Poor disintegration
- Misleading or insufficient product information
- Misleading or unsupported health claims

The rest of this chapter explains each problem and identifies the supplement types most susceptible to the problem. By being aware of

Common problems with supplements

Type of supplement	Common problems
Herbals	Too little or no active ingredient Wrong ingredient Contamination Misleading or unsupported health claims Dangerous or illegal ingredients
Vitamins	Too much active ingredient Poor disintegration Too little ingredient
Minerals	Too little or no active ingredient Poor disintegration
Special supplements	Too little or no active ingredient Contamination Misleading or insufficient product information
Traditional Chinese medicine*	Unexpected ingredients ("spiked" products)

* Note: Generally available only from special shops or practitioners of Chinese medicine

the problems, you'll know what to avoid when selecting certain supplements. (See Common problems with supplements, above.) Part 2 presents an indepth discussion of supplement types, the problems encountered with them, and tips for buying quality products.

Too little or no active ingredient

WHAT THIS MEANS
A product contains less of the main ingredient than the label indicates, or it's virtually devoid of that ingredient.

WHY THIS IS A PROBLEM
A product containing too little or no active ingredient is unlikely to perform as expected. This can cause you to think that an ingredient is ineffective. Or you could experience a change in your condition if you switch from a quality supplement to a version lacking sufficient active ingredient.

WHERE THIS IS MOST COMMON

Supplements made from expensive raw materials are most likely to contain less than the label indicates. Examples include SAMe, chondroitin, and some expensive herbals, such as saw palmetto. Products that can degrade over time, for example vitamin A, may also contain too little ingredient or no active ingredient. (Unfortunately, many supplements sit on store shelves for years.)

WHY THIS HAPPENS

If an ingredient is expensive, there's an economic incentive to put less of it in the bottle. Therefore, a manufacturer might skimp on using the ingredient, or the ingredient supplier might add fillers (with or without the manufacturer's knowledge). Although verifying ingredient quality should be standard practice for manufacturers — especially when materials are purchased at unusually low prices or are miraculously available when demand exceeds supply — many don't bother to check. Another possible reason for too little or no active ingredient is poor manufacturing practices. Measuring exact quantities for every pill requires sophisticated manufacturing skills, equipment, and quality-assurance procedures. Still another problem is product labeling. If the product's weight includes inactive materials to which the active ingredient is bound, then the labeled amount of active ingredient is misleading. (See "Misleading or insufficient ingredient information," page 17.)

HOW TO AVOID IT

Unfortunately, there's no easy way to tell if you're being short-changed on ingredients. But you can avoid products that may have degraded by checking expiration dates and selecting those with the most time left before expiration. And use ConsumerLab.com's list of quality products as a guide to the best supplements. (See "Part 2" and "Part 3.")

Too much active ingredient

WHAT THIS MEANS

A product has more active ingredient than is stated on the label.

WHY THIS IS A PROBLEM

Just because your body requires a certain amount of an ingredient doesn't mean that more is better. In fact for some products, most notably vitamins and minerals, upper limits (ULs) for tolerable intake have been established. If your intake is above the limit, you risk serious adverse effects. These ULs were established by the Institute of Medicine of the National Academy of Sciences. (See "Part 2.")

WHERE THIS IS MOST COMMON
This problem typically occurs with vitamins, minerals, and multivitamins. The reasons are twofold: the ingredients are relatively inexpensive and, in the case of the multis, measuring exact amounts for each ingredient is complex.

WHY THIS HAPPENS
Some manufacturers prefer to err on the side of using too much ingredient, particularly for ingredients that degrade over time. In addition, the Food and Drug Administration (FDA) requires that products contain the quantities listed but doesn't specify how much extra is allowed.

HOW TO AVOID IT
Compare the labels on supplements with the established ULs for the ingredients. Vitamins and minerals that now have ULs include vitamins A, B_6, C, D, and E; niacin; folate; choline; calcium; iron; phosphorus; iodine; magnesium; zinc; selenium; copper; manganese; and molybdenum. (See "Multivitamins & multiminerals," pages 33 to 53. Also see ConsumerLab.com's list of quality products in "Part 2" for a guide to the best supplements.)

Wrong ingredient

WHAT THIS MEANS
Nonherbal products rarely contain the wrong ingredient, but herbals commonly do. Specifically, herbal products may contain the wrong plant part or wrong species of plant. In addition, an herb or herbal extract should contain specific plant chemicals in the amounts shown to be most successful in clinical trials. Regrettably, growing, harvesting, and processing conditions, among other things, can easily affect these

chemicals. If, for example, the wrong species of herb or the wrong plant part is used or if the herb is harvested at the wrong time of year, the ingredient may be ineffective — or even dangerous.

WHY THIS IS A PROBLEM

If the ingredient used isn't the one known to be effective, the likelihood that the product will work is low. Furthermore, in some instances, the wrong ingredient—especially the wrong species or plant part in the case of herbs—can result in toxic effects.

WHERE THIS IS MOST COMMON

Herbal products, because of their complex nature, are the most likely supplements to contain the wrong ingredient. For example, in testing valerian products (an herbal sleep aid made from the root of the plant species Valeriana officinalis), ConsumerLab.com found some products that looked and smelled like valerian but lacked the chemical characteristics expected from the appropriate species.

WHY THIS HAPPENS

Some manufacturers don't carefully check the raw materials they receive from suppliers because they assume that the certificate of analysis that comes with the materials is correct. Manufacturers employing good quality control retest their materials before using them. In some instances, a manufacturer may accidentally purchase material of a different clinical quality. In this scenario, the fault may rest with the supplier who initially purchased material.

HOW TO AVOID IT

Learn the common and scientific names of herbs and other ingredients that you expect in a supplement. Sometimes a product claiming to have a certain herb, for example, will list a scientific name that doesn't match. Also, know which part of the herb is supposed to be used, and make sure that part is listed. This information should appear on a label's "Supplement Facts" panel. And use ConsumeLab.com's list of quality products as a guide to the best supplements. (See "Part 2" and "Part 3.")

Dangerous or illegal ingredients

WHAT THIS MEANS
Some ingredients found in supplements may be harmful even if the supplement is taken at the recommended dosage.

WHY THIS IS A PROBLEM
Some ingredients are toxic particularly to the liver and kidneys.

WHERE THIS IS MOST COMMON
Most ingredients cited as dangerous are herbal. Examples include aristolochic acid, which is found primarily in the plant Aristolochia and can cause kidney damage, and comfrey, which can cause liver toxicity. In April 2001, the FDA advised consumers not to use products containing aristolochic acid and asked manufacturers and distributors to recall such products. In July 2001, the FDA advised consumers to stop using comfrey products immediately and strongly recommended the industry remove such products from the market.

WHY THIS HAPPENS
Although the government bans proven-dangerous ingredients from use in supplements, manufacturers, not the government, are the ones primarily responsible for ensuring the safety of dietary supplements, according to the Dietary Supplement Health and Education Act (DSHEA). Manufacturers, therefore, should be aware of scientific reports of ingredient problems and take corrective steps. In practice, the FDA typically issues a warning before a manufacturer recalls a problem product.

HOW TO AVOID IT
Frequently check Recalls and Warnings on ConsumerLab.com's web site (http://www.consumerlab.com/recalls.asp) for FDA product warnings. And don't purchase or use ingredients with known problems. (See "Herbal alert," pages 21 to 26.)

Contamination

WHAT THIS MEANS

Besides wrong ingredients, products may contain chemicals or other materials that don't belong there. Possible contaminants include pesticides, microorganisms, heavy metals, manufacturing by-products, and even plants harvested accidentally.

WHY THIS IS A PROBLEM

Some contaminants can be toxic or carcinogenic, and their associated health problems can show up immediately—or in the future. Taking certain contaminated supplements for a short time may not pose much risk, but prolonged exposure will cause serious health risks. For example, toxins from mercury build up over time.

WHERE THIS IS MOST COMMON

Herbal products are most susceptible to pesticide contamination. For example, several Korean ginseng products that ConsumerLab.com tested contained heavy metals and two potentially toxic pesticides. But even synthetic products, such as creatine, aren't immune from contamination; they may be compromised by manufacturing by-products.

WHY THIS HAPPENS

Herbs can become contaminated in one of four ways. They may be:
- exposed to heavy metals and pesticides while growing (either intentionally or incidentally from cross-exposure to chemicals used in the soil or nearby)
- treated with pesticides—particularly fungicides, which prevent mold growth—during drying and preparation
- exposed to potentially dangerous pesticides that have banned from use on herbs in this country and then imported here
- accidentally contaminated with other herbs or plants harvested at the same time. In 1997, for example, large amounts of plantain were contaminated with Digitalis lanata, which can cause adverse cardiovascular reactions.

Poor manufacturing conditions may contribute to the contamination of nonherbal, synthetic supplements.

14

HOW TO AVOID IT
Use ConsumerLab.com's list of quality products as a guide to the best supplements. (See "Part 2.")

Unexpected ingredients ("spiked" products)

WHAT THIS MEANS
Although not a common practice, some supplements are spiked with ingredients not listed on their labels. Why add ingredients? To give a more pronounced effect.

WHY THIS IS A PROBLEM
Added ingredients can cause adverse reactions or interactions with other drugs or supplements. For competitive athletes, spiking can create additional problems as well. For example, many substances are banned from use during competition; if a banned substance is found in an athlete's blood or urine during routine testing, the athlete could be disqualified from competition.

WHERE THIS IS MOST COMMON
Spiking is most common in products where consumers expect an immediate effect. For example, ginseng, which is usually taken to increase vitality, may be spiked with caffeine, which is a stimulant. Creatine, which is used to increase endurance, may be spiked with the male hormone nandralone. But that isn't all. Traditional Chinese medicines are occasionally spiked with medicinal compounds that normally require a prescription. For example, diazepam, camphor, mercury, cannabis, codeine, prednisolone, aminopyrine, opium powder, arsenic, methyl salicylate, chlordiazepoxide, tetrahydropalmatine, methyltestosterone, and chloramphenicol have all been found.

WHY THIS HAPPENS
A manufacturer intentionally adds the ingredient to enhance the effect of the product. The intent is to keep the consumer buying the product because of its perceived helpful effect.

HOW TO AVOID IT

Avoiding spiked products is difficult. Supplements typically act as mild drugs. Therefore, if you experience very dramatic or adverse reactions from a supplement (especially if it's a traditional Chinese medicine), consider the possibility that it may be spiked with something more potent than the labeled ingredients. Because testing for every possible unlisted ingredient isn't feasible, even products passing ConsumerLab.com's evaluation may contain unidentified ingredients.

Poor absorption

WHAT THIS MEANS

To be useful, supplement ingredients must disintegrate and dissolve in the gut, then be absorbed and enter the bloodstream. The standard laboratory test for disintegration (formally known as the United States Pharmacopeia [USP] "Disintegration and Dissolution of Nutritional Supplements" method) attempts to mimic the conditions in the gut. During the test the product under investigation is continuously agitated in an acidic solution for up to 45 minutes. In that time, the pill should fall apart. Some manufacturers claim their products meet the USP specification, but the claim shouldn't be taken as certainty. The USP method was part of ConsumerLab.com's battery of tests for evaluating products.

WHY THIS IS A PROBLEM

Pills that don't disintegrate properly can't dissolve and be absorbed; they will simply pass through the body unused.

WHERE THIS IS MOST COMMON

Poor disintegration is most common with vitamin and mineral supplements. However, other products, including herbals, sold in tightly packed tablets or caplets can remain intact after the 45-minute acid test. Most capsules, by contrast, fall apart easily, and most chewable products — as long as they're chewed—disintegrate.

WHY THIS HAPPENS

Poor disintegration usually results from poor manufacturing practices and quality control.

HOW TO AVOID IT

Use ConsumerLab.com's list of quality products as a guide to the best supplements. (See "Part 2" and "Part 3.")

To determine for yourself your supplement's ability to disintegrate, try the following test (it isn't foolproof, but it does yield helpful information): Heat $1/2$ cup of vinegar in a heat-safe cup on the hot-plate portion of a coffee machine to 98.6° F (body temperature). For a quick check of the temperature, use an instant-read thermometer, and don't allow it to rest on the bottom of the cup where heat is most intense, giving a false reading. If necessary, move the cup on and off the heat to maintain a constant temperature. Place a pill in the cup, then stir continuously for 30 to 45 minutes, without hitting the pill. Uncoated or shiny thinly coated products should disintegrate before the maximum time; gelatin and hard-coated products will require the full time. Note: This test may not work with time-release products. And be aware that chewable products are meant to be broken down by chewing. Remember, this test isn't as rigorous as a laboratory test, but it is more accurate than simply dropping the supplement into cold vinegar.

Misleading or insufficient ingredient information

WHAT THIS MEANS

The name used to describe the ingredient(s) is misleading.

WHY THIS IS A PROBLEM

The product may have far less of the active ingredient expected.

WHERE THIS IS MOST COMMON

Typically, misleading information appears in three situation: (1) Products that claim to be special "formulas," "blends," or "complexes" may be hiding information. For example, ConsumerLab.com discovered that the product "Pyruvate 1000," whose label indicated that it contained 1,000 mg of a "pyruvate formula," contained only about 250 mg pyruvate. (2) Another fairly common but confusing tactic is to use unfamiliar chemical names. For example, the weight of an ingredient may include inactive materials to which the active ingredient is bound.

These inactive ingredients are typically sugars or salts and may account for as much as half of the claimed weight of the active material. For example, the active molecule in SAMe is S-adenosyl-methionine and the non-active part of SAMe may be "1,4-butanedisulfonate" or "tosylate disulfate." Therefore, if the non-active parts are included in the weight of SAMe in the "Supplement Facts" panel on the product, only about half the amount is active SAMe. Chemical names are commonly used for SAMe, glucosamine, and isoflavones from soy products. (3) Confusion also arises when products are marketed under the chemical names for natural and synthetic ingredients. Unfortunately, natural and synthetic products vary not only in chemical names but also in activity levels. Vitamin E is a good example here. It takes more synthetic vitamin E (dl-alpha-tocopherol) to achieve the same therapeutic level as natural vitamin E (d-alpha-tocopherol).

WHY THIS HAPPENS

Sometimes a manufacturer is reluctant to share a propriety formula, so the label may simply say "formula," "blend," or "complex," without stating ingredient quantities. Other times, a manufacturer wants to save money by using less of the active ingredient.

HOW TO AVOID IT

Learn about supplement ingredients, and be wary of names that include added terms such as salts. Also, be cautious if a term such as formula, blend, or complex appears on the label's "Supplement Facts" panel. Use ConsumerLab.com's list of quality products as a guide to the best supplements. (See "Part 2" and "Part 3.")

Misleading or unsupported health claims

WHAT THIS MEANS

Some supplement labels make unsupported health claims. Others may show health claims for ingredients not in the product.

WHY THIS IS A PROBLEM

By making promises (via health claims) that they can't keep, some supplement manufacturers entice consumers to purchase unproven products — a step that may cause the consumer to delay getting much-needed medical treatment.

WHERE THIS IS MOST COMMON

Misleading or unsupported health claims can appear on any product. However, products claiming to be "special formulas" lend themselves most easily to deceptive advertising by unscrupulous manufacturers. After all, such claims can't be readily verified, disproved, or compared to other products.

WHY THIS HAPPENS

Products can sport unsupported health claims because no government agency reviews labels for accuracy or truthfulness before marketing. After a product is on the market, the Federal Trade Commission (FTC) will try to correct errors or stop untruthful advertising if a problem is brought to the agency's attention. For example in 2001, the FTC fined a Utah herbal supplement company $100,000 for advertising that a comfrey supplement could cure a wide range of diseases, including asthma, arthritis, and cancer. The FTC said the claims had no scientific information to back them up.

HOW TO AVOID IT

Learn as much as you can about product ingredients and the results of clinical studies. Be aware that most supplements aren't allowed to state that they can "treat" or "prevent" disease. (Only over-the-counter or prescription drugs can normally make such claims.)

As of the end of 2001, the FDA has allowed only 13 claims regarding the ability of certain nutrients or foods to prevent or treat specific diseases. Most permitted FDA claims relate to broad dietary changes, not to the consumption of single nutrients. None of the approved claims relate to herbal ingredients.

But to confuse matters, the FDA considers numerous health-related statements to be "structure or function claims," not health claims, and the agency hasn't reviewed, denied, or approved them. Such function claims include "vitamin C provides antioxidant protection," "garlic helps maintain healthy serum-cholesterol levels," and "saw palmetto helps maintain a healthy prostate."

A health claim on a supplement label is typically an abbreviated form of the FDA-approved claim. Be wary of products that specifically claim to prevent or treat diseases, but don't contain the specified ingredients. (See FDA-approved claims, below.)

FDA-approved claims

Ingredient	Approved health claim
Calcium	Regular exercise and a healthy diet with enough calcium help teen and young adult white and Asian women maintain good bone health and may reduce their risk of osteoporosis.
Sodium	Diets low in sodium may reduce the risk of high blood pressure, a disease associated with many factors.
Fat	Development of cancer depends on many factors. A diet low in total fat may reduce the risk of some cancers.
Saturated fat and cholesterol	While many factors affect heart disease, diets low in saturated fat and cholesterol may reduce the risk of this disease.
Fiber	Low-fat diets rich in fiber-containing grain products, fruits, and vegetables may reduce the risk of some types of cancer, a disease associated with many factors.
Fruits, vegetables, and grain products that contain fiber, particularly soluble fiber	Diets low in saturated fat and cholesterol and rich in fruits, vegetables, and grain products that contain some types of dietary fiber, particularly soluble fiber, may reduce the risk of some types of cancer, a disease associated with many factors.
Fruits and vegetables	Low-fat diets rich in fruits and vegetables (foods that are low in fat and may contain dietary fiber, vitamin A, or vitamin C) may reduce the risk of some types of cancer, a disease associated with many factors.
Folate	Healthful diets with adequate folate may reduce a woman's risk of having a child with brain or spinal cord birth defect.
Potassium	Diets containing foods that are good sources of potassium and low in sodium may reduce the risk of high blood pressure and stroke.
Sugar alcohols	Frequent between-meal consumption of foods high in sugars and starches promotes tooth decay. The sugar alcohols in this food do not promote tooth decay.
Soluble fiber in whole oats and psyllium	Diets low in saturated fat and cholesterol that include 3 grams of soluble fiber from whole oats per day may reduce the risk of heart disease.
Soy protein	Diets low in saturated fat and cholesterol that include 25 grams of soy protein a day may reduce the risk of heart disease.
Whole grains	Diets rich in whole grain foods and other plant foods and low in total fat, saturated fat, and cholesterol may reduce the risk of heart disease and certain cancers.

CHAPTER 3

Herbal alert

Some supplements, especially herbals, can interfere with prescription drugs and anesthesia. Other herbals are toxic and best avoided altogether. This chapter discusses interactions as well as potentially harmful ingredients.

Interactions with drugs

Numerous herbal supplements can interfere with the action of certain prescription drugs and either lessen or amplify their effectiveness, leading to underdosing, overdosing, and other problems. For example, St. John's wort can compromise the effects of several drugs, including birth control drugs and drugs for heart disease, seizures, and cancer, according to a Food and Drug Administration (FDA) public health advisory. And the popular herb ginkgo can amplify the effects of warfarin, increasing the risk of bleeding. The risks associated with such interactions are both dose related and high, so be sure to inform your physician if you're using a supplement.

Interactions with anesthesia

Herbal supplements can also interact with anesthesia. The American Society of Anesthesiologists has warned that some herbs can cause problems with heart rate, blood pressure, and bleeding when combined with anesthesia. Some of the most popular herbs are of greatest concern, including St. John's wort, ginkgo biloba, and ginseng. Because an informed physician can better manage potential interactions, the Society recommends alerting your anesthesiologist if you use a supplement as well as not taking it for 2 to 3 weeks before surgery, if possible. (See "Cautions and concerns" in "Part 2.")

12 Potentially hazardous ingredients

Although many herbals are safe and effective, the following 12 are potentially toxic. For updates as new information is released, visit Recalls and Warnings on ConsumerLab.com's web site (http://www.consumerlab.com/recalls.asp).

ARISTOLOCHIC ACID
Aristolochia is found in herbal supplements for treating arthritis, allergies, prostatitis, circulation problems, and weight loss. The herb produces aristolochic acid, a toxin that can cause cancer and end-stage kidney failure. The FDA has stated that any botanical containing aristolochic acid is considered unsafe and adulterated. Plants in these species, among others, may be contaminated with aristolochia, according to the FDA: Akebia, Asarum, Bragantia, Clematis, Cocculus, Diploclisia, Menispermum, Mu Tong, Sinomenium, Soussurea lappa, Stephania, and Vladimiria souliei.

BUTCHER'S BROOM
Butcher's broom, also called broom, is promoted mainly as a treatment for improving circulation in the legs. Broom contains toxic alkaloids and hydroxytyramine and shouldn't be used except under close medical supervision. Large doses can cause vomiting, purging, rapid heart rate, and low blood pressure. Advanced stages of toxicity can cause complete collapse of the respiratory system. Large doses have been reported to cause fatal poisoning.

CHAPARRAL
Commonly called the creosote bush, chaparral is a desert shrub historically used by Native Americans for treating various ailments—

most commonly for "cleansing" the blood and correcting skin conditions. In the early 1990s, authorities identified several cases of chaparral-related liver disease, two of which resulted in liver failure requiring transplants. At the time, chaparral products were removed from the shelves, and today, most major retailers don't carry them, but the products are available on the Internet. Overdosing with chaparral capsules is easy.

COLTSFOOT

The dried leaves or flowers of Tussilago farfara L. used to be a popular remedy for treating coughs and bronchial congestion. However, researchers discovered that all parts of the plant contain a compound that's toxic to the liver, and animal studies have shown that rats fed diets containing coltsfoot develop cancerous liver tumors. Because hot water easily extracts the toxic compound, health-safety experts advise against using teas as well as capsules.

COMFREY

Historically, comfrey has been used as a blood purifier and a treatment for stomach ulcers. Applied topically, comfrey is supposed to aid the healing of broken bones and wounds. Herbal supplements that contain Symphytum officionale (common comfrey), S. asperum (prickley comfrey), or S. x uplandicum (Russian comfrey) are sources of pyrrolizidine alkaloids, which are toxic to the liver and other tissues. Several incidences of liver disease and liver failure in people who regularly consumed comfrey tea or supplements have also been reported in scientific literature. The FDA issued an advisory asking supplement manufacturers to remove comfrey products from the market. However, some products are still available.

EPHEDRA

Also known as ma huang, ephedra is a natural source of ephedrine alkaloids, compounds that have amphetamine-like (stimulant) effects. Although ephedra is common in weight-loss products, it can cause a wide variety of adverse reactions, including nervousness, anxiety, irregular heartbeat, hypertension, insomnia, psychosis, seizures, heart attack, and stroke; it can even cause death. Therefore, people who have diabetes, glaucoma, heart disease, high blood pressure, thyroid disease, impaired circulation in the brain, an enlarged prostate, or kidney problems should avoid taking it. Ephedra is also contraindicated in people taking ephedrine alkaloids, such as some cold medicines, or monoamine oxidase inhibitors. The FDA currently recommends consuming no more than 8 mg of ephedra alkaloids per dose and less than 24 mg/day. Unfortunately, determining ephedra intake is difficult because the amount in an herbal preparation may not be clearly or accurately stated on the label.

In January 2002, the Canadian government requested a voluntary recall of products containing either ephedra or ephedrine after concluding that these products pose a serious health risk. The products in the recall include ephedra and ephedrine products that have a dose unit of more than 8 mg of ephedrine or a label recommending more than 8 mg/dose or 32 mg/day or that recommend or imply that they're to be used for more than 7 days; all combination products containing ephedra or ephedrine together with stimulants (such as caffeine) and other ingredients that might increase the effect of ephedra or ephedrine in the body; and ephedra or ephedrine products with labeled or implied claims for appetite suppression, weight loss, metabolic enhancement, increased exercise tolerance, body-building effects, euphoria, increased energy or wakefulness, or other stimulant effects. Products containing ephedra that are marketed for traditional medicine will continue to be available, provided they don't contain caffeine and the ephedrine content doesn't exceed 8 mg/dose or more than 32 mg/day. A product that combined large doses of ephedrine with caffeine has been reported as a contributing factor in one death in Canada.

GERMANDER

Wild germander (Teuchrium chamaedrys L.), which has been marketed in Europe as a weight-loss aid, is used in medicinal teas, elixirs, capsules, and tablets, and sometimes in combination with other herbs. The herb has been linked to a number of cases of serious liver disease and at least one death. Recent research suggests that liver disease induced by germander may be caused by both a direct toxicity on the liver and immune reactions that damage the liver. France prohibited the use of germander several years ago, and other countries currently restrict its use. Germander isn't commonly found in the United States, but it could show up in imported herbal products or products purchased from overseas online.

KAVA

Kava (Piper methysticum) is promoted for relaxation (that is, to relieve stress, anxiety, and tension), sleeplessness, and menopausal symptoms. The FDA has received several reports of liver-related injuries as well as a report of a previously healthy young female who required a liver transplant after consuming kava. In March 2002, the FDA advised that kava-containing dietary supplements posed a risk of severe liver injury, including hepatitis, cirrhosis, and liver failure. Germany, Switzerland, France, Canada, the United Kingdom, and several other countries have warned consumers about the potential risks of kava use as well. Some countries have also removed kava-containing products from the marketplace.

Given these reports, those who have liver disease or liver problems or who are taking a drug that can affect the liver should consult a physician before using a supplement that contains kava. Consumers who use a kava-containing supplement and experience signs of liver disease should also consult their physician. Signs of serious liver disease include jaundice (yellowing of the skin or whites of the eyes) and brown urine. Nonspecific signs and symptoms include nausea, vomiting, light-colored stools, unusual tiredness, weakness, stomach or abdominal pain, and loss of appetite.

Commonly used names for kava include ava, ava pepper, awa, intoxicating pepper, kava, kava kava, kava pepper, kava root, kava-kava, kawa, kawa kawa, kawa-kawa, kew, Piper methysticum, P. methysticum Forst.f., P. methysticum G. Forst., rauschpfeffer, sakau, tonga, wurzelstock, and yangona.

PENNYROYAL

Pennyroyal comes from two members of the mint family: Hedeoma pulegiodes L. Pers., the American pennyroyal, and Mentha pulegium L., the European pennyroyal. The herb is promoted as a stimulant, a treatment for gas, and a way to promote menstrual flow or induce abortion. Only lethal or near-lethal doses can induce abortion. More than 20 cases of pennyroyal toxicity from brewed teas and small amounts of the oil have been reported.

SCULLCAP

Although scullcap is promoted as being an overall tonic with tranquilizing and antispasmodic effects, no proof exists that scullcap has any therapeutic value. It has, however, been associated with some cases of poisoning. What's unclear is whether the poisoning was from scullcap or from adulteration with germander, which is sometimes mistaken or substituted for scullcap.

WORMWOOD

Better known as absinthe, wormwood (Artemisia absinthium L.) contains a pleasant-smelling but toxic oil that contains the compound thujone. The herb is best known as the main flavoring ingredient in the strong, green-colored alcoholic beverage called absinthe. The drink was popular in the early 1900s until researchers discovered its mind-altering, addictive, and toxic effects, and it was outlawed in most countries. As a medicinal herb, the dried leaves, flowers, and essential oil of wormwood have been used to treat cancer and intestinal worms, improve blood circulation, and stimulate the heart. Although it's still available in teas, tinctures, and capsules, wormwood is extremely toxic and isn't recommended under any circumstances.

YOHIMBE

Yohimbe is a tree bark containing a variety of pharmacologically active chemicals. Sometimes referred to as an herbal Viagra, yohimbe is generally found in products for men and is said to aid body building and sexual performance. However, the FDA has received reports of yohimbe's serious adverse effects, including renal failure, seizures, and death. The major active compound in yohimbe is yohimbine, a chemical that causes blood vessels to dilate, thereby lowering blood pressure. At high doses, yohimbine acts as a monoamine oxidase inhibitor and causes serious adverse reactions if taken with foods rich in tyramine (such as liver, aged cheeses, red wine, and overripe bananas) or with over-the-counter drugs containing phenylpropanolamine, an ingredient used in some nasal decongestants. The FDA recommends that people with low-blood pressure, diabetes, or heart, liver, or kidney disease avoid yohimbe. Signs and symptoms of overdose include weakness and nervous stimulation followed by paralysis, fatigue, stomach disorders, and possibly death.

CHAPTER 4

Product testing

This chapter provides an overview of ConsumerLab.com's selection and testing process for the vitamins and minerals, herbal products, and special dietary supplements appearing in the product reviews. (See "Part 2" and "Part 3.")

Selection and testing

For its product reviews, ConsumerLab.com selected the supplements most commonly sold in the United States and chose samples from a wide variety of brands. None of the products for testing were obtained directly from the manufacturer. However, manufacturers and distributors were given the opportunity to request testing of their products, either through ConsumerLab.com's Guaranteed Testing Program (products were tested along with those selected by ConsumerLab.com) or through ConsumerLab.com's Ad Hoc Testing Program (products were tested after the initial, large review). Companies paid a fee for testing on request. They weren't, however, allowed to send samples for testing, nor could they specify the lot to be tested. All products were purchased through retail stores, on-line retailers, catalogs, health care professionals, or multilevel marketing companies.

Testing methods

For each of the reviews in this book, ConsumerLab.com evaluated the products using the best testing methods and standards available. Consequently, many of the tests surpassed the requirements of the U.S. Food and Drug Administration. We tested all products to determine whether they contained the main ingredient specified on the label. On supplements known to have specific problems, we performed additional tests. For example, some reports indicate that ginseng may be contaminated with pesticides, so we tested that particular herb for those chemicals. Also, calcium and iron products may be contaminated with lead, so we checked those products for that contaminant. In addition, we tested many products in tablet form for disintegration. (See "Poor absorption," pages 16 to 17.) Specific testing methods are detailed in individual product reviews.

Passing standards

For a product to pass ConsumerLab.com's evaluations, it had to meet specific criteria in either a first or second round of testing. Passing scores in each analysis included margins of technical error. In addition, ConsumerLab.com reserved the right to disqualify a product at any time if it seemed to be unsafe or to provide misleading or inaccurate label information.

The CL seal

Manufacturers whose products meet ConsumerLab.com's standards can license the flask-shaped CL Seal of Approved Quality Products for use on labels and in promotional materials. To ensure continuing compliance with ConsumerLab.com's standards, products are periodically reevaluated.

How to read ConsumerLab.com s product seal

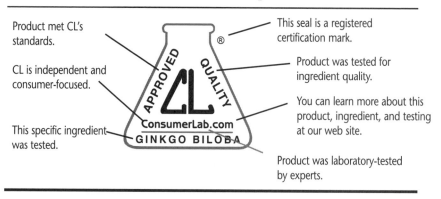

Product met CL's standards.

CL is independent and consumer-focused.

This specific ingredient was tested.

This seal is a registered certification mark.

Product was tested for ingredient quality.

You can learn more about this product, ingredient, and testing at our web site.

Product was laboratory-tested by experts.

Product updates

It's routine practice for manufacturers to discontinue products, change product ingredients, and alter information about their products. Therefore, when purchasing a supplement, read labels carefully. If a product's ingredients differ from those reviewed in this book, the product may be of a different quality than the one tested. Remember, too, that all products from a manufacturer or distributor aren't necessarily of equal quality.

Other information you should know:

• Products that aren't listed here either weren't tested or failed testing.

• Manufacturers may ask ConsumerLab.com to evaluate additional products, and if the products pass our tests, we will add them to the web site and to future editions of this book.

• Additional information about products can be found in the back of this book. (See "More brand information," page 191, and "On-line resources," page 207.)

PART TWO

Product reviews for vitamins and minerals

Multivitamins & Multiminerals

WHAT IT IS

Multivitamins and multiminerals, collectively referred to as multis, are the most popular dietary supplements in America. But for consumers, what's in a multi can be confusing because the ingredients vary widely by brand and even within brands. Part of the reason for variation is no established standard. Still three factors make establishing a standard difficult:

- Supplementation needs vary because people's diets differ.
- Recommended intakes of specific vitamins and minerals established by the Institute of Medicine of the National Academies vary according to age, gender, and health status.
- Some health care professionals advocate dosages that differ from the Institute of Medicine's recommendations.

The Institute of Medicine has issued many new and revised recommendations in the past few years, including a major update on January 9, 2001. However, the U.S. Food and Drug Administration (FDA), still doesn't require manufacturers to include this new information in the "% Daily Value" that appears in "Supplement Facts" on product labels. Even when the FDA requires the information or a manufacturer reformulates a product, it may be years before consumers see the changes because supplements commonly remain on shelves for years.

WHAT IT DOES

Multivitamins are generally used as "nutrition insurance" — that is, to fill nutrition gaps in dietary intake. Although a well-balanced diet can meet the recommended intakes for all nutrients, nutrition surveys have repeatedly shown that most people's diets are low in several nutrients. Some studies have also found that people who regularly take multivitamins have stronger immune systems and possibly a lowered risk of age-related cognitive decline.

QUALITY CONCERNS

Because no government agency is responsible for routinely testing multivitamin and multimineral supplements for their contents or quality, ConsumerLab.com independently evaluated several of the leading multivitamin and multimineral products to determine four things:

- whether they possess the ingredient types and amounts stated on their labels
- whether they disintegrate readily
- whether they're free from impurities
- whether they compare favorably with the most recently recommended Dietary Reference Intakes (DRIs).

PRODUCT TESTING

ConsumerLab.com purchased 27 brands of multivitamin and multimineral products: 15 general multis (no specified age or gender category, but evaluated only for adult use), 2 prenatal multis, 3 women's multis, 2 senior's multis (generally for people ages 50 and older), and 5 children's multis. These products were tested for their amounts of several common labeled ingredients: folic acid, calcium, and vitamin A (retinol and beta-carotene). Because not all products were labeled to contain every one of these ingredients, some products were alternatively tested for other ingredients—for example, vitamin C (ascorbic acid) if folic acid wasn't an ingredient, and iron or zinc if calcium wasn't an ingredient. Products were also tested for disintegration (excluding chewable and time-release products), lead contamination, and compliance with the most recent DRIs. (See "ConsumerLab.com's testing methods and standards," page 169.)

TEST FINDINGS

Of the 27 products that ConsumerLab.com tested, 9 products, or one-third, failed to meet the criteria for the product review. This failing group was made up of 5 general, 2 women's, 1 prenatal, and 1 children's product. Both senior's products passed.

The reasons the products failed the evaluation were as follows:

Vitamin A: The most common problems were related to vitamin A. One children's product, for example, had more than 150% of its labeled vitamin A (as retinol), giving it the equivalent of more than 7,000 IUs (International Units) per tablet, which is in excess of the recently established Tolerable Upper Intake Levels (ULs) for children as well as adults.

Another two products (a general and a women's product) had less than 40% of their labeled beta-carotene. The women's product also didn't meet its label claim for total vitamin A.

One general multi had more than its stated beta-carotene, but less than half of its stated vitamin A from retinol.

Disintegration: One general multi failed to disintegrate properly, suggesting that its contents wouldn't be fully available for use in the body.

Folic Acid and Vitamin C: One prenatal product had 75% of its stated folic acid, a vitamin thought to reduce the risk of certain birth defects. One general multi had only 50% of its claimed folic acid. At the other end of the spectrum, another general multi had more than 165% of its labeled folic acid. Too much folic acid can mask the early signs of anemia from vitamin B_{12} deficiency, especially in the elderly. (Vitamin B_{12} deficiency, if untreated, can lead to irreversible nerve damage.) Only one product tested didn't claim to have folic acid and was, therefore, tested for ascorbic acid (vitamin C), for which it met its claimed amount.

Calcium, Zinc, and Iron: All but four products claimed to contain calcium, and one general multi had more than 150% of the claimed amount. The four products without calcium were tested for iron or zinc and contained those nutrients in claimed amounts. Niacin: High levels of niacin can cause skin flushing as well as tingling, itching, burning, and pain. Although these signs and symptoms aren't life threatening, the UL for adults is 35 mg/day. The RDA for men is 16 mg and for women 14 mg. Four general multis (one of which also failed on other criteria) claimed levels of 50 to 100 mg per suggested daily serving, exceeding the UL. One women's product also exceeded the UL.

Lead: No product exceeded the contamination levels for lead. In fact, all products had less than 0.5 mcg of lead per serving—well below the safe limit of 3 mcg used by ConsumerLab.com and the state of California.

In addition, four products were considered conditionally approved because they passed laboratory analyses for content but exceeded the ULs for specific vitamins and minerals. This group included three children's products that exceeded the ULs for copper, niacin, vitamin A, or zinc for certain young age-groups and one adult general-use product that exceeded the UL for niacin if taken at the upper range of its suggested dosage.

QUALITY PRODUCTS

Listed alphabetically by name on page 37 are the products that passed ConsumerLab.com's independent testing of multivitamin and multimineral supplements (see Multivitamin and multimineral conditionally approved products, pages 37 to 38, and Multivitamin and multimineral approved-quality products, pages 39 to 45).

CONSUMERTIPS™ FOR BUYING AND USING

ConsumerLab.com has prepared numerous important tips about dosing, selecting, and buying multivitamin and multimineral supplements. This information—along with our list of approved-quality brands—provides a valuable guide for choosing appropriate products.

As required by the FDA, dietary supplement labels or packaging must state the "% of Daily Value" for each vitamin and mineral the product contains. However, not all percentages given

Multivitamins and multiminerals conditionally approved products

These products passed ConsumerLab.com's laboratory testing for quality. However, some ingredients exceeded the upper levels (ULs) of tolerable intake for certain individuals.

General

Ocuvite® Zinc with Key Antioxidants Vitamin and Mineral Supplement (tablet)

Dist: Bausch & Lomb® Pharmaceuticals, Inc.

Acceptable only at 1 tablet/day. Label suggests 1 to 2 tablets; taking more than 1 tablet exceeds UL for zinc.

Vitamin A (100% as beta-carotene) 5,000 I.U.; Vitamin C (ascorbic acid) 60 mg; Vitamin E (dl-alpha tocopherol acetate) 30 I.U.; Zinc (from zinc oxide) 40 mg; Selenium (from sodium selenate) 40 mcg; Copper (from cupric oxide) 2 mg

---

Puritan's Pride One® Long Acting Multivitamin and Mineral Supplement (tablet)*

Mf: Puritan's Pride. Inc.

Slightly exceeds UL for Niacin

Vitamin A (as retinyl palmitate and beta-carotene) 10,000 I.U.; Vitamin C (as ascorbic acid with rose hips) 250 mg; Vitamin D (as cholecalciferol) 400 I.U.; Vitamin E (as d-Alpha Tocopheryl Acetate) 30 I.U.; Thiamin (vitamin B1, as thiamine hydrochloride) 25 mg; Riboflavin (Vitamin B2); Niacin (as niacinamide) 50 mg; Vitamin B6 (as pyridoxine hydrochloride) 50 mg; Folic Acid 400 mcg; Vitamin B12 (as cyanocobalamin) 50 mcg; Biotin (as d-Biotin) 50 mcg; Pantothenic Acid (as d-calcium pantothenate) 50 mg; Calcium (as bonemeal) 50 mg; Iron (as ferrous fumarate) 10 mg; Phosphorus (as bonemeal) 23 mg; Iodine (as potassium iodide) 150 mcg; Magnesium (as magnesium oxide) 100 mg; Zinc (as zinc sulfate) 15 mg; Selenium (as selenium yeast) 25 mcg; Copper (as copper sulfate) 2 mg; Manganese (as manganese sulfate) 5 mg; Chromium (as chromium chloride) 100 mcg; Molybdenum (as sodium molybdate) 15 mcg; Chloride (as potassium chloride) 1 mg;

(continued)

Children's

Potassium (as potassium chloride) 1 mg; PABA (para-aminobenzoic acid) 50 mg; Inositol 15 mg; Choline Bitartrate 15 mg

Flintstones® Plus Iron Children's Multivitamin Plus Iron Supplement (chewable tablet)

Dist: Bayer Corp.

Acceptable only for children ages 4 and older; levels of niacin and vitamin A exceed ULs for younger children.

Vitamin A 2,500 IU; Vitamin C 60mg; Vitamin D 400 I.U.; Vitamin E 15 I.U.; Thiamin (B1) 1.05 mg; Riboflavin (B2) 1.2mg; Niacin 13.5 mg; Vitamin B6 1.05 mg; Folic Acid 300 mcg; Vitamin B12 4.5 mcg; Iron (elemental) 15mg

---

Spring Valley® Children's Chewables Complete with Beta Carotene & Essential Minerals (chewable tablet)

Leiner Health Products

Acceptable only for children ages 9 and older; levels of zinc exceed ULs for younger children.

Vitamin A 5,000 I.U. (50% as beta-carotene); Vitamin C 60 mg; Vitamin D 400 I.U.; Vitamin E 30 I.U.; Thiamin (Vitamin B1) 1.5 mg; Riboflavin (Vitamin B2) 1.7 mg; Niacin 20 mg; Vitamin B6 2 mg; Folate 400 mcg; Vitamin B12 6mcg; Biotin 40 mcg; Pantothenic Acid 10 mg; Calcium 100 mg; Iron 18 mg; Phosphorus 100 mg; Iodine 150 mcg; Magnesium 20 mg; Zinc 15 mg; Copper 2 mg; Sodium 10 mg

---

Sundown® Pokemon™ Complete Children's Multiple Vitamin and Mineral Supplement (chewable tablet)

Sundown Vitamins

Acceptable only for children ages 9 and older; levels of copper, niacin, vitamin A, and zinc exceed ULs for younger children.

Total Carbohydrate <1g; Sugars <1g; Sorbitol <1g; Vitamin A 5,000 I.U.; Vitamin C (as sodium ascorbate and ascorbic acid) 60 mg; Vitamin D (as cholecalciferol) 400 I.U.; Vitamin E (as dl-alpha tocopheryl acetate) 30 I.U.; Thiamin (Vitamin B1)(as thiamin mononitrate) 1.5 mg; Riboflavin (Vitamin B2) 1.7 mg; Niacin (as niacinamide) 20 mg; Vitamin B6 (as pyridoxine HCl) 2 mg; Folic Acid 400 mcg; Vitamin B12 (as cyanocobalamin) 6 mcg; Biotin 40 mcg; Pantothenic Acid (as calcium d-pantothenate) 10 mg; Calcium 150 mg; Iron (as ferrous sulfate) 18 mg; Phosphorus 80 mg; Iodine (as potassium iodide) 150 mcg; Magnesium (as magnesium oxide) 20 mg; Zinc (as zinc oxide) 15 mg; Copper (as cupric oxide) 2 mg

---

* Tested through ConsumerLab.com's Ad Hoc Testing Program (Product was tested at the manufacturer's request after the initial review was completed and released.)

‡ See "More Brand Information," page 191.

Multivitamin and multimineral approved-quality products

Note: Not all products state the chemical form of each ingredient.

General (Evaluated for adult use)

Geritol Complete® High Potency Multi-Vitamin Plus Multi-Mineral Dietary Supplement (tablet)

Dist: SmithKline Beecham Consumer Healthcare

Vitamin A 7,250 I.U. (100% as Beta-Carotene); Vitamin C 60 mg; Vitamin D 400 I.U.; Vitamin E 30 I.U.; Vitamin K 30 mcg; Thiamine (Vitamin B_1) 1.7 mg; Riboflavin (Vitamin B_2) 1.7 mg; Niacin 20 mg; Vitamin B_6 2.5 mg; Folic Acid 0.42 mg; Vitamin B_{12} 6.7 mg; Biotin 0.045 mg; Pantothenic Acid 14 mg; Calcium 154 mg; Iron 16 mg; Phosphorus 120 mg; Iodine 120 mcg; Magnesium 95 mg; Zinc 13.5 mg; Copper 1.8 mg; Manganese 2.5 mg; Chromium 13 mcg; Molybdenum 10 mcg; Selenium 1 mcg; Chloride 25 mg; Potassium 36 mg

Kirkland Signature™ Daily Multi-Vitamin/Mineral Dietary Supplement (tablet)

Dist: CWC, Inc.

Vitamin A 10,000 I.U. (25% as Beta-Carotene); Vitamin C 120 mg; Vitamin D 400 I.U.; Vitamin E 60 I.U.; Vitamin K 25 mcg; Thiamin (Vitamin B1) 1.5 mg; Riboflavin (Vitamin B2) 1.7 mg; Niacin 20 mg; Vitamin B_6 2 mg; Folate (Folic Acid) 400 mcg; Vitamin B_{12} 6 mcg; Biotin 30 mcg; Pantothenic Acid 10mg; Calcium 162 mg; Iron 9 mg; Phosphorus 109 mg; Iodine 150 mcg; Magnesium 100 mg; Zinc 22.5 mg; Selenium 45 mcg; Copper 3 mg; Manganese 2.5 mg; Chromium 100 mcg; Molybdenum 25 mcg; Chloride 36.3 mg; Sodium Less than 5 mg; Potassium 40 mg; Nickel 5 mcg; Tin 10 mcg; Silicon 2 mg; Vanadium 10 mcg; Boron 150 mcg

Life Essentials® Dietary Supplement (capsule)

Mfd. for Pharmanex, Inc.

Vitamin A (as Vitamin A Palmitate, 29% as Beta-Carotene from Dunaliella Salina) 3,500 I.U.; Vitamin C (as Ascorbic Acid, Acerola Cherry Extract) 70 mg; Vitamin D3 (as Cholecalciferol) 200 I.U.; Vitamin E (as D-Alpha Tocopheryl Succinate; and Beta, Gamma, and Delta Tocopherols) 30 I.U.; Thiamin (as Thiamine Mononitrate) 0.75 mg; Riboflavin (as Riboflavin) 0.85 mg; Niacin (as Niacinamide) 10 mg; Vitamin B_6 (as Pyridoxine Hydrochloride, Pyridoxal-5-Phosphate) 1 mg; Folate (as Folic Acid) 200 mcg; Vitamin B_{12} (as Cyanocobalamin) 3 mcg; Biotin (as Biotin) 75 mcg; Pantothenic Acid (as D-Calcium Pantothenate) 5 mg; Calcium (as Calcium Carbonate, Calcium Chelate) 100 mg; Iron (as Iron Chelate) 1.5 mg; Iodine (as Potassium Iodide) 37.5 mcg; Magnesium (as Magnesium Chelate, Magnesium Citrate, Magnesium Oxide) 50 mg; Zinc (as Zinc Chelate) 7.5 mg; Selenium (as L-Selenomethionine) 17.5 mcg; Copper (as Copper Chelate) 1 mg; Manganese (as Manganese Chelate) 1.75 mg; Chromium (as Chromium Chelate) 60 mcg; Molybdenum (as Molybdenum Chelate) 37.5 mcg; Potassium (as Potassium Chloride) 40 mg; Boron (as Boron Citrate) 0.5 mg;

(continued)

Horsetail Extract 75 mg

Nature Made® Essential Balance® Complete High Potency Multi Vitamin/Mineral Supplement (tablet)* ‡

Dist: Nature Made

Vitamin A 5,000 I.U.; Vitamin C 120 mg; Vitamin D 400 I.U.; Vitamin E 50 I.U.; Vitamin K 25 mcg; Thiamin 1.5 mg; Riboflavin 1.7 mg; Niacin 20 mg; Vitamin B_6 2 mg; Folate 400 mcg; Vitamin B_{12} 6 mcg; Biotin 30 mcg; Pantothenic Acid 10 mg; Calcium 100 mg; Iron 9 mg; Phosphorus 77 mg; Iodine 150 mcg; Magnesium 100 mg; Zinc 15 mg; Selenium 25 mcg; Copper 2 mg; Manganese 2 mg; Chromium 120 mcg; Molybdenum 25 mcg; Chloride 36 mg; Potassium 40 mg; Boron 150 mcg; Nickel 5 mcg; Tin 10 mcg; Vanadium 10 mcg; Lutein 250 mcg

Nature's Bounty® Multi-Day™ Multivitamin Supplement with Beta Carotene Dietary Supplement (tablet)*

Mf: Nature's Bounty, Inc.

Vitamin A (as Retinyl Acetate and Beta-Carotene) 5,000 I.U.; Vitamin C (as Ascorbic Acid) 60 mg; Vitamin D (as Cholecalciferol) 400 I.U.; Vitamin E (as dl-Alpha Tocopheryl Acetate) 10 I.U.; Thiamin (Vitamin B_1) (as Thiamine Mononitrate) 1.5 mg; Riboflavin (Vitamin B_2) 1.7 mg; Niacin (as Niacinamide) 20 mg; Vitamin B_6 (as Pyridoxine Hydrochloride) 2 mg; Folic Acid 400 mcg; Vitamin B_{12} (as Cyanocobalamin) 6 mcg; Pantothenic Acid (as d-Calcium Pantothenate) 10 mg

Nature's Bounty® Nutritional Support for Your Skin, Hair, & Nails Dietary Supplement (tablet)*

Mf: Nature's Bounty, Inc.

Vitamin A (as Retinyl Palmitate) 1667 I.U.; Vitamin C (as Ascorbic Acid and Rose Hips) 20 mg; Vitamin D (as Cholecalciferol) 33.3 I.U.; Vitamin E (as d-Alpha Tocopheryl Acetate) 5 I.U.; Thiamin (Vitamin B_1) (as Thiamine Mononitrate) 1.67 mg; Riboflavin (Vitamin B_2) 1.67 mg; Niacin (as Niacinamide) 8.3 mg; Vitamin B_6 (as Pyridoxine Hydrochloride) 1.67 mg; Folic Acid 66.7 mcg; Vitamin B_{12} (as Cyanocobalamin) 2.67 mcg; Biotin (as D-Biotin) 66.7 mcg; Pantothenic Acid (as D-Calcium Pantothenate) 5 mg; Calcium (as Dicalcium Phosphate and Calcium Carbonate) 278 mg; Iron (as Ferrous Gluconate) 1 mg; Phosphorus (as Dicalcium Phosphate) 110 mg; Iodine (as Potassium Iodide) 37.5 mcg; Magnesium (as Magnesium Oxide) 33.3 mg; Zinc (as Zinc Gluconate) 2.5 mg; Selenium (as Sodium Selenate) 4.2 mcg; Manganese (as Manganese Gluconate) 1.67 mg; PABA (Para-Aminobenzoic Acid) 8.3 mg; Choline Bitarate 25 mg; Inositol 10 mg; RNA 10 mg; Citrus Bioflavonoids 8.3 mg; Rutin 4.2 mg; Betaine Hydrochloride 8.3 mg; Rose Hips 20 mg

Nature's Bounty® Vitamin ABC Plus™ Multi-vitamin and Multi-Mineral Formula Dietary Supplement (tablet)*

Mf: Nature's Bounty, Inc.

Vitamin A (as Retinyl Acetate and Beta-Carotene) 5,000 I.U.; Vitamin C (as Ascorbic Acid) 60 mg; Vitamin D (as Cholecalciferol) 400 I.U.; Vitamin E (as dl-Alpha Tocopheryl Acetate) 30 I.U.; Vitamin K (as Phytonadione) 25 mcg; Thiamin (Vitamin B_1) (as Thiamine Mononitrate) 1.5 mg; Riboflavin (Vitamin B_2) 1.7 mg; Niacin (as Niacinamide) 20 mg; Vitamin B_6 (as Pyridoxine Hydrochloride) 2 mg; Folic Acid 400 mcg; Vitamin B_{12} (as Cyanocobalamin) 6 mcg; Biotin (as D-Biotin) 30 mcg; Pantothenic Acid (as D-Calcium Pantothenate) 10 mg; Calcium (as Dicalcium Phosphate and Calcium Carbonate) 162 mg; Iron (as Ferrous Fumarate) 18 mg; Phosphorus (as Dicalcium Phosphate) 109 mg; Iodine (as Potassium Iodide) 150 mcg; Magnesium (as Magnesium Oxide) 100 mg; Zinc (as Zinc Oxide) 15 mg; Selenium (as Sodium Selenate) 20 mcg; Copper (as Cupric Oxide 2 mg; Manganese (as Manganese Sulfate) 3.5 mg; Chromium (as Chromium Chloride) 65 mcg; Molybdenum (as Sodium Molybdate) 160 mcg; Chloride (as Potassium Chloride) 80 mcg; Boron (as Sodium Borate) 150 mcg; Nickel (as Nickel Sulfate) 5 mcg; Tin (as Stannous Chloride) 10 mcg; Silicon (as Sodium Metasilicate and Silicon Dioxide) 2 mg; Vanadium (as SodiumMetavanadate) 10 mcg

Nutrilite® Daily Multivitamin and Multimineral Dietary Supplement (tablet)‡

Access Business Group International LLC

Vitamin A (20% as Beta-Carotene) 5,000 I.U.; Vitamin C 90 mg; Vitamin D 400 I.U.; Vitamin E 30 I.U.; Vitamin K 80 mcg; Thiamin 2.3 mg; Riboflavin 2.6 mg; Niacin 20 mg; Vitamin B_6 2 mg; Folic Acid 400 mcg; Vitamin B_{12} 9 mcg; Biotin 300 mcg; Pantothenic Acid 10 mg; Calcium 200 mg; Iron 6 mg; Phosphorus 45 mg; Iodine 150 mcg; Magnesium 100 mg; Zinc 15 mg; Selenium 70 mcg; Copper 2 mg; Manganese 2 mg; Chromium 120 mcg; Molybdenum 75 mcg; Nutrilite® concentrate 518 mg

Nutrilite® Double X Multivitamin Multimineral (tablet)*‡

Access Business Group International LLC

One Serving (one Gold, one Silver, one Bronze tablet) contains: Vitamin A (from DOUBLE X Concentrate) (75% as natural Beta-Carotene) 5,000 I.U.; Vitamin C (from Ascorbic Acid, Acerola Powder and DOUBLE X Concentrate) 250 mg; Vitamin D (from DOUBLE X Concentrate) 200 I.U.; Vitamin E (from DOUBLE X Concentrate, d-Alpha Tocopheryl Succinate) 150 I.U.; Vitamin K (from Phytonadione) 40 mcg; Thiamin (from DOUBLE X Concentrate) 12.5 mg; Riboflavin (from DOUBLE X Concentrate) 12.5 mg; Niacin (from DOUBLE X Concentrate) 35 mg; Vitamin B_6 (from DOUBLE X Concentrate) 25 mg; Folic Acid (from DOUBLE X Concentrate) 400 mcg; Vitamin B_{12} (from DOUBLE X Concentrate) 50 mcg; Biotin (from d-Biotin) 150 mcg; Pantothenic Acid (from DOUBLE X Concentrate) 25 mg; Calcium (from Calcium Carbonate) 450 mg; Phosphorus (from Calcium Phosphate) 10 mg; Iodine (from DOUBLE X Concentrate) 75 mcg; Magnesium (from Magnesium Oxide) 225 mg; Zinc (from Zinc Gluconate) 10 mg; Selenium (from Sodium Selenite) 50 mcg; Copper (from Copper Gluconate) 1 mg; Manganese (from Manganese Gluconate) 2.5 mg; Chromium (from Chromium Chloride) 60 mcg; Molybdenum (from Sodium Molybdate) 37.5 mcg; Potassium (from Potassium Chloride and DOUBLE X Concentrate)

(continued)

40 mg; Alpha Lipoic Acid (from DOUBLE X Concentrate) 5 mg; MSM (Methylsulfonyl Methane) (from DOUBLE X Concentrate) 30 mg; Lycopene (from DOUBLE X Concentrate) 0.5 mg; Lutein (from DOUBLE X Concentrate) 0.5 mg; Quercetin (from DOUBLE X Concentrate) 50 mg; Spirulina (from DOUBLE X Concentrate) 25 mg; Boron (from Boron Aspartate) 500 mcg; Vanadium (from Vanadyl Sulfate) 10 mcg; DOUBLE X Concentrate (AWP concentrate—Alfalfa Extract [leaf, stem], Watercress Dehydrate [leaf, stem], Parsley Dehydrate [leaf, stem], Acerola Concentrate [*Malphigia glabra*] [fruit], Citrus Bioflavonoid Concentrate [grapefruit, mandarin, lemon] [whole fruit and peel], Quercitin, Methylsulfonyl Methane, Brassica Concentrate—Broccoli [*Brassica oleracea*] [floret], Horseradish [*Amoracia rusticana*] [root], Mixed tocopheryls, Calcium Pantothenate, Pyridoxine Hydrochloride, Niacinamide, Spirulina [*Arthrospira plateneis*] [algae], Thiamine Mononitrate, Riboflavin; Alpha-Lipoic Acid, Beta-Carotene, Niacin, Lutein, Lycopene, Vitamin A Acetate, Folic Acid, Potassium Iodide, Vitamin B12, Vitamin D3, Magnesium Oxide)

One A Day Maximum Multivitamin/Multimineral Supplement (tablet)

Dist: Bayer Corp

Vitamin A 5,000 I.U.; Vitamin C 60 mg; Vitamin D 400 I.U.; Vitamin E 30 I.U.; Vitamin K 25 mcg; Thiamin (B_1) 1.5 mg; Riboflavin (Vitamin B_2) 1.7 mg; Niacin 20 mg; Vitamin B_6 2 mg; Folate 400 mcg; Vitamin B_{12} 6 mcg; Biotin 30 mcg; Pantothenic Acid 10 mg; Calcium (elemental) 162 mg; Iron 18 mg; Phosphorus 109 mg; Iodine 150 mcg; Magnesium 100 mg; Zinc 15 mg; Selenium 20 mcg; Copper 2 mg; Manganese 3.5 mg; Chromium 65 mcg; Molybdenum 160 mcg; Chloride 72 mg; Potassium 80 mg; Boron 150 mcg; Nickel 5 mcg; Silicon 2 mg; Tin 10 mcg; Vanadium 10 mcg

SynerPro® Multiple Vitamins and Minerals, Vitamin and Mineral Supplement with SynerPro® Concentrate (tablet)

Dist: Nature's Sunshine Products, Inc.

Vitamin A (Beta-Carotene) 2,500 I.U.; Vitamin C 30 mg; Vitamin D (Fish Oils) 200 I.U.; Vitamin E (d-Alpha Tocopherol) 15 I.U.; Thiamine (Vitamin B_1) 0.75 mg; Riboflavin (Vitamin B_2) 0.85 mg; Niacin (as Nicotinic Acid) 10 mg; Vitamin B_6 (Pyridoxine HCl) 1 mg; Folate (Folic Acid) 200 mcg; Vitamin B_{12} (Cyanocobalamin) 3 mcg; Biotin 150 mcg; Pantothenic Acid (d-Calcium Pantothenate) 5 mg; Calcium (d-Calcium Pantothenate and Dicalcium Phosphate) 125 mg; Iron (Ferrous Fumarate) 9 mg; Phosphorus (Dicalcium Phosphate) 90 mg; Iodine (Potassium Iodide) 75 mcg; Magnesium (Magnesium Oxide) 50 mg; Zinc (Zinc Oxide) 7.5 mg; Selenium (Amino Acid Chelate) 25 mcg; Copper (Copper Gluconate) 1 mg; Manganese (Amino Acid Chelate) 0.5 mg; Chromium (Amino Acid Chelate) 50 mcg; Molybdenum (Amino Acid Chelate) 38 mcg

Theragran-M® Advanced Multivitamin/Multimineral Supplement, High Potency Formula (caplet)

Mfd. for Bristol-Myers Products

Vitamin A 5,000 I.U. (20% as Beta-Carotene); Vitamin C 90 mg; Vitamin D 400 I.U.; Vitamin E 60 I.U.; Vitamin K 28 mcg; Thiamin 3 mg (Vitamin B1); Riboflavin 3.4 mg (Vitamin B_2); Niacin 20 mg; Vitamin B_6 6 mg; Folate 400 mcg; Vitamin B_{12} 12 mcg; Biotin 30 mcg; Pantothenic Acid 10 mg; Calcium 40 mg; Iron 9 mg; Phosphorus 31 mg; Iodine 150 mcg; Magnesium 100 mg; Zinc 15 mg; Selenium 70 mcg; Copper 2 mg; Manganese 2 mg; Chromium 50 mcg; Molybdenum 75 mcg; Chloride 7.5 mg; Potassium 7.5 mg; Boron 150 mcg; Nickel 5 mcg; Silicon 2 mg; Tin 10 mcg; Vanadium 10 mcg

Vita-Smart® High Potency Vitamins and Minerals Confirmed Release Dietary Supplement (tablet)

Dist: Kmart

Vitamin A 8,000 I.U.; Vitamin C 120 mg; Vitamin D 400 I.U.; Vitamin E 30 I.U.; Thiamin 5 mg; Riboflavin 5 mg; Niacin 30 mg; Vitamin B_6 5 mg; Folic Acid 400 mcg; Vitamin B_{12} 10 mcg; Biotin 10 mcg; Pantothenic Acid 10 mg; Calcium 100 mg; Iron 18 mg; Phosphorus 78 mg; Iodine 150 mcg; Magnesium 100 mg; Zinc 15 mg; Copper 2 mg; Chloride 15 mg; Potassium 15 mg

Walgreens Multiple Vitamins with Iron One Daily for Adults and Children, Dietary Supplement (tablet)

Dist: Walgreen Co.

Vitamin A 5,000 I.U.; Vitamin C 60 mg; Vitamin D 400 I.U.; Vitamin E 30 I.U.; Thiamin (Vitamin B_1) 1.5 mg; Riboflavin (Vitamin B_2) 1.7 mg; Niacin 20 mg; Vitamin B_6 2 mg; Folate 400 mcg; Vitamin B_{12} 6 mcg; Pantothenic Acid 10 mg; Iron 18 mg

Prenatal

Stuart Prenatal® Multivitamin/Multimineral Supplement (tablet)

Dist: Integrity Pharmaceutical Corp (formally marketed by Wyeth Laboratories Inc.)

Vitamin A 4,000 I.U. (25% as Beta-Carotene); Vitamin C 100 mg; Vitamin D 400 I.U.; Vitamin E 11 mg; Thiamin 1.8 mg; Riboflavin 1.7 mg; Niacin 18 mg; Vitamin B_6 2.6 mg; Folic Acid 0.8 mg; Vitamin B_{12} 4 mcg; Calcium 200 mg; Iron 27 mg; Zinc 25 mg

Women's

Safeway Select Women's One Tablet Daily Plus Calcium, Iron & Zinc Dietary Supplement, Multivitamin/Multimineral (tablet)

Dist: Safeway, Inc.

Vitamin A 5,000 I.U. (50% as Beta-Carotene); Vitamin C 60 mg; Vitamin D 400 I.U.; Vitamin E 30 I.U.; Thiamin (Vitamin B_1) 1.5 mg; Riboflavin (Vitamin B_2) 1.7 mg; Niacin 20 mg; Vitamin B_6 2 mg; Folate 400 mcg; Vitamin B_{12} 6 mcg; Pantothenic Acid 10 mg; Calcium 450 mg; Iron 27 mg; Zinc

 (continued)

Men's

15 mg

Vitamin World™ High Potency Time Release Ultra Vita Man® Vitamin, Mineral & Herb Formula for Men Dietary Supplement (tablet)*

Mf: Vitamin World

Vitamin A (as Retinyl Palmitate) 2,500 I.U.; Vitamin C (as Ascorbic Acid and Rose Hips) 150 mg; Vitamin D (as Cholecalciferol) 100 I.U.; Vitamin E (as d-Alpha Tocopheryl Acetate) 50 I.U.; Vitamin K (as Phtonadione) 12.5 mcg; Thiamin (Vitamin B_1) (as Thiamine Mononitrate) 15 mg; Riboflavin (Vitamin B_2) 15 mg; Niacin (as Niacinamide) 15 mg; Vitamin B_6 (as Pyridoxine Hydrochloride) 15 mg; Folic Acid 200 mcg; Vitamin B_{12} (as Cyanocobalamin) 15 mcg; Biotin (as D-Biotin) 150 mcg; Pantothenic Acid (as D-Calcium Pantothenate) 15 mg; Calcium (as Calcium Carbonate and Calcium Phosphate) 137.5 mg; Phosphorus (as Dicalcium Phosphate) 105 mg; Iodine (as Potassium Iodide) 75 mcg; Magnesium (as Magnesium Oxide) 50 mg; Zinc (as Zinc Gluconate) 25 mg; Selenium (as Sodium Selenate) 12.5 mcg; Copper (as Copper Gluconate) 1 mg; Manganese (as Manganese Gluconate) 2.5 mg; Chromium (as Chromium Picolinate) 25 mcg; Potassium (as Potassium Chloride) 15 mg; Choline (as Choline Bitarate) 5 mg; Inositol 5 mg; PABA (Para-Aminobenzoic Acid) 5 mg; L-Cystenine (as L-Cystenine Hydrochloride) 50 mg; Silica (as Silicon Dioxide) 10 mg; Citrus Bioflavonoids 12.5 mg; Super Oxide Dismutase (SOD from Bovin Liver Extract) 5 mcg; Pycnogenol® Pine Bark Extract (Pinus maritima) 0.5 mcg; Yohimbe Bark Extract (*Pausinystalia yohimbe*) 25 mg; Korean Ginseng Root (*Panax ginseng*) 25 mg; Oat Straw (*Avena sativa*) 25 mg; Damiana Leaf (*Turnera diffusa*) 25 mg; Muira Puama Bark (*Liriosma ovata*) 25 mg; Nettle Leaf (*Urtica dioica*) 15 mg; Oyster Extract 12.5 mg; Saw Palmetto Berry (*Serenoa repens*) 25 mg; Prostate Glandular 25 mg; Pumpkin Seed (*Curcurbita pepo*) 15 mg; Golden Seal Root (*Hydrastis canadensis*) 12.5 mg; Pygeum Bark (*Pygeum africanum*) 12.5 mg; Proprietary Herbal Blend 12.5 mg, Cayenne Pepper Fruit (*Capsicum frutescens*), Alfalfa Leaf (*Medicago sativa*), Garlic Bulb (*Allium sativum*); Lecithin, Oat Bran (*Avena sativa*), Parsley Leaf (*Petroselinum crispum*), Sarsaparilla Root (*Smilax*

Senior's

AARP Pharmacy Service Formula 502 Seniors Vitamins and Minerals Supplement, USP (caplet)

Dist: Retired Persons Services, Inc

Vitamin A (as vitamin A acetate and 3% as Beta-Carotene) 5,200 I.U.; Vitamin C (as Ascorbic Acid) 60 mg; Vitamin D (as Cholecalciferol) 200 I.U.; Vitamin E (as dl-Alpha Tocopheryl Acetate) 15 I.U.; Thiamin (Vitamin B_1 as Thiamine Mononitrate) 1.2 mg; Riboflavin (Vitamin B2) 1.4 mg; Niacin (as Niacinamide) 16 mg; Vitamin B6 (as Pyridoxine Hydrochloride) 2.2 mg; Folic Acid (Folate) 400 mcg; Vitamin B_{12} (as Cyanocobalamin) 3 mcg; Pantothenic Acid (as d-Calcium Pantothenate) 10 mg; Calcium (as Dicalcium Phosphate and Calcium Carbonate) 100 mg; Iron (as Ferrous Fumarate) 10 mg; Phosphorus (as Dicalcium Phosphate) 77 mg; Iodine (as Potassium Iodide) 150 mcg; Magnesium (as Magnesium Oxide) 30 mg; Zinc (as Zinc Oxide) 15 mg; Copper (as Cupric Sulfate)

44

2 mg; Manganese (as Manganese Sulfate) 1 mg; Potassium (as Potassium Sulfate) 5 mg

Centrum® Silver® Specially Formulated Multivitamin Multimineral Dietary Supplement for Adults 50+ (tablet)‡

Dist: Whitehall-Robins Healthcare

Vitamin A 5,000 I.U. (20% as Beta-Carotene); Vitamin C 60 mg; Vitamin D 400 I.U.; Vitamin E 45 I.U.; Vitamin K 10 mcg; Thiamin 1.5 mg; Riboflavin 1.7 mg; Niacin 20 mg; Vitamin B_6 3 mg; Folic Acid 400 mcg; Vitamin B_{12} 25 mcg; Biotin 30 mcg; Pantothenic Acid 10 mg; Calcium 200 mg; Phosphorus 48 mg; Iodine 150 mcg; Magnesium 100 mg; Zinc 15 mg; Selenium 20 mcg; Copper 2 mg; Manganese 2 mg; Chromium 150 mcg; Molybdenum 75 mcg; Chloride 72 mg; Potassium 80 mg; Boron 150 mg; Nickel 5 mg; Silicon 2 mg; Vanadium 10 mcg; Lutein 250 mcg

Children's

Poly-Vi-Sol® Chewable Vitamins and Minerals with Iron, Peter Rabbit™ Shapes (chewable tablet)
(*Note:* Label states not for children younger than age 4)

Dist: Mead Johnson Nutritionals

Vitamin A 2,500 I.U.; Vitamin C 60 mg; Vitamin D 400 I.U.; Vitamin E 15 I.U.; Thiamin 1.05 mg; Riboflavin 1.2 mg; Niacin 13.5 mg; Vitamin B6 1.05 mg; Folate 0.3 mg; Vitamin B_{12} 4.5 mcg; Iron 12 mg; Zinc 8 mg; Copper 0.8 mg

* Tested through the ConsumerLab.com's Ad Hoc Testing Program (Product was tested at the manufacturer's request after the initial review was completed and released.)
‡ See "More Brand Information," page 191.

reflect the latest Recommended Dietary Allowances (RDAs) or Adequate Intakes (AIs). What's more, the products aren't required to indicate whether their ingredients exceed the Tolerable Upper Intake Levels (ULs) for their target audience. Unfortunately, many do exceed these ULs. (See Understanding Recommended Dietary Allowances, Adequate Intakes, Tolerable Upper Intake Levels.)

Most products state an amount for each claimed ingredient. To help you determine whether such amounts are appropriate for you, we've listed the RDAs, AIs, and ULs for vitamins and minerals as appropriate. Remember that 1,000 mcg (micrograms) equals 1 mg (milligram), and 1,000 mg equals 1 gram. IU stands for International Units and is used for those ingredients measured by their biological activity rather than weight.

Understanding Recommended Dietary Allowances, Adequate Intakes, Tolerable Upper Intake Levels

Recommended Dietary Allowances (RDAs), Adequate Intakes (AIs), and Tolerable Upper Intake Levels (ULs), established by the Institute of Medicine of the National Academies, are collectively known as DRIs.

An RDA is the average daily dietary intake level that's sufficient to meet the nutrient requirement of nearly all healthy individuals of a particular life stage and gender. An AI, similar to an RDA, is an approximation used when there isn't enough information to develop an RDA. A UL is the maximum amount of a nutrient that most people can take in on a daily basis, without posing a risk of adverse health effects. As intake increases above the UL, the risk of adverse reactions also increases. Like the RDAs and AIs, the ULs vary according to age, life stage, and gender. Individuals shouldn't regularly exceed the UL without medical recommendation and supervision.

THE VITAMINS

VITAMIN A

Vitamin A is necessary for maintaining good vision and skin. In supplements, vitamin A usually refers to retinol (including retinyl palmitate and retinyl acetate) and beta-carotene. Retinol is found in animal-derived sources, such as dairy foods and liver. Beta-carotene comes from fruits and vegetables, such as carrots and spinach, and is converted in the body to vitamin A, based on the body's need; therefore, it may be the safest form of vitamin A. Although supplement labels generally combine beta-carotene and retinol when calculating vitamin A content, many also note the percentage of vitamin A that comes from beta-carotene. People who rely on beta-carotene as their primary source of vitamin A, such as vegetarians, should note that recent evidence shows beta-carotene has only half the vitamin A activity previously believed. Vitamin A is usually indicated in IUs. Labels may alternatively (and actually more correctly) list their vitamin A content in micrograms, though it may be expressed in milligrams. For vitamin A, 1 microgram equals 3,333 IUs.

Recommended intake: The RDA is 1,000 IU for children ages 1 to 3; 1,333 IU for children ages 4 to 8; and 2,000 IU for children ages 9 to 13. For males ages 14 and older, the RDA is 3,000 IU. For females ages 14 and older, it's 2,333 IU. These amounts can be obtained from food.

Upper limit: Too much vitamin A can be toxic. The effects of vitamin A toxicity include abnormalities in the liver, central nervous system, bone, and skin. These abnormalities also apply to the offspring of pregnant or breast-feeding women. Newly established ULs specify that daily intake shouldn't exceed 2,000 IU for children ages 1 to 3; 3,000 IU for children ages 4 to 8; 5,666 IU for children ages 9 to 13; 9,333 IU for teens ages 14 to 18; and 10,000 IU for adults. However, these ULs apply only to vitamin A consumed from supplements, fortified foods, and animal sources; they don't include vitamin A consumed as beta-carotene or from fruits and vegetables.

Supplements may exceed the newly released ULs, particularly those products designed to meet the needs of a broad age range of individuals, such as children's vitamins.

B VITAMINS

Detailed information on the B vitamins can be found in the section on that topic (see "B Vitamins [Thiamin, Riboflavin, Niacin, Pantothenic Acid, B_6, Folic Acid, B_{12}, and Biotin]," pages 54 to 69).

VITAMIN C

Detailed information on the vitamin C can be found in the section on that topic (see "Vitamin C," pages 70 to 75).

VITAMIN D

Vitamin D (cholecalciferol) helps the body absorb calcium for strong bones and teeth. It can be obtained in sufficient amounts from fortified milk and foods as well as from exposure to sunlight. (Note: Dark-skinned individuals absorb less light because of skin pigmentation and are somewhat more likely to be vitamin D deficient).

Vitamin D is measured as micrograms of cholecalciferol or in IUs of vitamin D activity. For vitamin D, 1 mcg equals 40 IUs.

Recommended intake: An AI has been established but is only relevant if an individual isn't getting adequate exposure to sunlight. The AI is 5 mcg (200 IU) for individuals ages 1 to 50, 10 mcg (400 IU) for individuals ages 51 to 70, and 15 mcg (600 IU) for individuals ages 71 and older.

Upper limit: Too much vitamin D can result in hypercalcemia (too much calcium in the blood) with signs and symptoms including high blood pressure, irregular heartbeat, nausea, and seizures. Taking too much during pregnancy can cause abnormalities in the fetus. The UL for individuals ages 1 and older is 50 micrograms (2,000 IU).

VITAMIN E

Detailed information on the vitamin E can be found in the section on that topic (see "Vitamin E," pages 76 to 81).

VITAMIN K

Vitamin K plays a role in blood clotting and may strengthen bones. Foods, such as green leafy vegetables, can provide sufficient amounts.

Recommended intake: The AI for vitamin K is measured in micrograms (shown as mcg). The AI is 30 mcg for children ages 1 to 3, 55 mcg for children ages 4 to 8, 60 mcg for children ages 9 to 13, and 75 mcg for teens ages 14 to 18. For males, ages 19 and older, the AI is 120 mcg. For females ages 19 and older, it's 90 mcg.

Upper Limit: No UL has been established for vitamin K.

THE MINERALS

CALCIUM

Calcium, which is critical for strong bones and teeth, is a bulky material and therefore, most multis don't contain the recommended daily intake because the tablet would be quite large. Consequently, calcium supplements or fortified foods or beverages are better supplement sources.

Detailed information on calcium can be found in the section on that topic (see "Calcium," pages 82 to 89).

CHROMIUM

Chromium helps regulate blood sugar levels and may reduce the risk of diabetes. Chromium is found in liver, cheese, eggs and whole-wheat products, but many Americans may be deficient.

Recommended intake: Chromium is typically expressed in micrograms (mcg), though supplement labels may list it as milligrams (mg). The AI is 11 mcg for children ages 1 to 3 and 15 mcg for children ages 4 to 8. For males ages 9 to 13, the AI is 25 mcg; for females, it's 21 mcg. For males ages 14 to 50, it's 35 mcg. For females ages 14 to 18, it's 24 mcg, increasing to 25 mcg for females ages 19 to 50. For males ages 51 older, it's 30 mcg; for females ages 51 and older, it's 20 mcg. For pregnant women, the AI is 29 mcg if they're younger than age 18 and 30 mcg if they're age 19 or older. For breast-feeding women, the AI is 44 mcg if they're younger than age 18 and 45 mcg if they're age 19 or older.

Upper limit: No UL has been established for chromium.

COPPER

Copper is necessary for proper development of connective tissue, nerve coverings, and skin pigment and is found in organ meats, oysters, nuts, seeds and fortified cereals. It can be obtained in sufficient quantity from a varied diet.

Animal studies show that copper oxide (or cupric) may not be well absorbed. Copper sulfate, cupric acetate, and alkaline copper carbonate are, therefore, preferable alternatives. Unfortunately, copper oxide is common in supplements because it's less bulky and allows for smaller pills.

Recommended intake: Copper in supplements may be shown in milligrams (mg) or micrograms (mcg). The RDA is 340 mcg for children ages 1 to 3, 440 mcg for ages 4 to 8, 700 mcg for children ages 9 to 13, 890 mcg for teens ages 14 to 18. For adults ages 19 years and older, the RDA is 900 mcg. For pregnant women, the RDA is 1,000 mcg; for breast-feeding women, it's 1,300 mcg.

Upper limit: Excessive consumption of copper may cause nausea and liver damage. The daily UL for copper is 1,000 mcg for children ages 1 to 3; 3,000 mcg for children ages 4 to 8; 5,000 mcg for children ages 9 to 13; 8,000 mcg for teens ages 14 to 18; and 10,000 mcg for adults ages 19 and older.

IODINE

Iodine is needed for making thyroid hormones. Deficiency can cause mental retardation, hypothyroidism, goiter, and dwarfism. Other than some seafood, most foods don't provide much iodine; most table salt, however, is iodized and represents a good dietary source of iodine.

Recommended intake: Iodine is typically measured in micrograms (mcg), though it's sometimes expressed in milligrams (mg). The RDA is 90 mcg for children ages 1 to 8 and 120 mcg for children ages 9 to 13. For both males and females ages 14 and older, the RDA is 150 mcg. For pregnant women, it's 220 mcg; for breast-feeding women, it's 290 mcg. Too much iodine taken during pregnancy can cause problems such as abnormal thyroid function in infants.

Upper limit: ULs for iodine are 200 mcg for children ages 1 to 3, 300 mcg for children ages 4 to 8, 600 mcg for children ages 9 to 13, 900 mcg for teens ages 14 to 18, and 1,100 mcg for adults ages 19 and older.

IRON

Iron deficiency is the leading cause of anemia and is most common in menstruating woman; it's also seen in some children and pregnant women. Meat, poultry, and fish are rich in iron. Dried fruits, grains, and green leafy vegetables are also good sources, although iron from plant sources is absorbed only half as well as that from animal sources.

Detailed information on iron can be found in the section on that topic (see "Iron," pages 90 to 95).

MAGNESIUM

Magnesium assists metabolism and is essential for the nervous system. Most of the daily requirement can be obtained from whole grains, fortified cereals, spinach, peanut butter, and beans.

Recommended intake: The RDA is 80 mg for children ages 1 to 3, 130 mg for children ages 4 to 8, and 240 mg for children ages 9 to 13. For males ages 14 to 18, the RDA is 410 mg; for males ages 19 to 30, 400 mg; and for males ages 31 and older, 420 mg. For females ages 14 to 18, it's 360 mg; for females ages 19 to 30, 310 mg; and for females ages 31 and older, 320 mg. For pregnant women younger than age 18, it's 400 mg; for those ages 19 to 30, 350 mg; and for those ages 31 and older, 360 mg. For breast-feeding women younger than age 18, it's 360 mg; for those ages 19 to 30, 310 mg; and for those age 31 or older, 320 mg.

Upper limit: Too much magnesium can cause diarrhea, nausea and vomiting, low blood pressure, and muscle weakness. The UL for magnesium applies only to supplements or other medication and is 65 mg for children ages 1 to 3 and 110 mg for children ages 4 to 8. For individuals ages 9 and older, the UL is 350 mg. It may seem inconsistent that the ULs are lower than the RDAs mentioned in the paragraph above. The reason is that magnesium from food sources doesn't cause the adverse reactions that magnesium from supplements does.

MANGANESE

Manganese is involved in bone formation and metabolism. Nuts, legumes, tea, and whole grains are rich sources of manganese and can provide adequate amounts.

Recommended intake: The AI for manganese is 1.2 mg for children ages 1 to 3 and 1.5 mg for children ages 4 to 8. For males ages 9 to 13, the AI is 1.9 mg; for males ages 14 to 18, 2.2 mg; and for males ages 19 and older, 2.3 mg. For females ages 9 to 18, it's

1.6 mg; for females age 19 or older, 1.8 mg. For pregnant women, it's 2.0 mg/day; for breast-feeding women, it's 2.6 mg/day.

Upper limit: Too much manganese may have adverse neurological effects. The UL for manganese is 2 mg for children ages 1 to 3, 3 mg for children ages 4 to 8, 6 mg for children ages 9 to 13, and 9 mg for teens ages 14 to 18. The UL for adults ages 19 and older is 11 mg.

Individuals with liver disease may experience adverse reactions at a lower level of manganese intake than the general population, and vegetarians may have significant manganese intake (10 to 20 mg/day) from their diets from nuts, legumes, tea, and whole grains. Adverse neurological effects, similar to symptoms caused by Parkinson's disease, have been observed in individuals who have consumed high amounts of manganese over time. Iron absorption by the gut may also be inhibited by high magnesium intake.

MOLYBDENUM

Molybdenum enhances various body enzymes and can be obtained from legumes, grain products, and nuts. Deficiency is rare in the United States.

Recommended intake: RDA for molybdenum is given in micrograms, though it's sometimes expressed in milligrams. The RDA is 17 mcg for children ages 1 to 3, 22 mcg for children ages 4 to 8, 34 mcg for children ages 9 to 13, and 43 mcg for teens ages 14 to 18. For adults ages 19 older, it's 45 mcg/day. For pregnant or breast-feeding women, it's 50 mcg/day.

Upper limit: Massive amounts of molybdenum can cause gout-like symptoms. The UL for molybdenum is 300 mcg for children ages 1 to 3; 600 mcg for children ages 4 to 8; 1,100 mcg for children ages 9 to 13; 1,700 mcg for teens ages 14 to 18; and 2,000 mcg for adults ages 19 and older.

SELENIUM

Selenium acts as an antioxidant and may help prevent cancer and heart damage in selenium-deficient individuals. Foods containing selenium include nuts, wheat germ, whole wheat, and orange juice. Many people don't get sufficient selenium from their diets.

Recommended intake: The RDA is 20 mcg for children ages 1 to 3 years, 30 mcg for children ages 4 to 8, and 40 mcg for children ages 9 to 13. For individuals ages 14 and older, the RDA is 55 mcg. For pregnant women, it's 60 mcg; for breast-feeding women, it's 70 mcg.

Upper limit: At very high doses, selenium can cause hair loss and tissue damage. The UL for selenium is 90 mcg for children ages 1 to 3, 150 mcg for children ages 4 to 8, and 280 mcg for children ages 9 to 13. The UL for adults ages 19 and older is 400 mcg.

ZINC

Zinc plays a role in brain function, wound healing, and sperm production. Many breakfast cereals are fortified with zinc, and it's naturally abundant in red meats, certain seafood, and whole grains. However, mild zinc deficiency is fairly common.

Recommended intake: The RDA of zinc is 3 mg for children ages 1 to 3, 5 mg for children ages 4 to 8, and 8 mg for children ages 9 to 13. For males ages 14 and older, the RDA is 11 mg. For females ages 14 to 18, it's 9 mg. For adults ages 19 and older, it's 8 mg/day. For pregnant women younger than age 18, the RDA is 13 mg; for pregnant women ages 19 and older, it's 11 mg. For breast-feeding women younger than age 18, the RDA is 14 mg; for breast-feeding women ages 19 and older, it's 12 mg.

Upper limit: Too much zinc can impair the absorption of copper and potentially depress the immune system. Recently established ULs for zinc are 7 mg for children ages 1 to 3, 12 mg for children ages 4 to 8, 23 mg for children ages 9 to 13, 34 mg for teens ages 14 to 18, and 40 mg for adults ages 19 and older.

B Vitamins
(Thiamin, Riboflavin, Niacin, Pantothenic Acid, B_6, Folic Acid, B_{12}, and Biotin)

WHAT IT IS
There are eight B vitamins — individually known as thiamin (B_1), riboflavin (B_2), niacin (B_3), pantothenic acid (B_5), pyridoxine (B_6), folic acid (folate), cyanocobalamin (B_{12}), and biotin. Like most vitamins, B vitamins are essential — your body can't make them; you must get them from your diet or from supplements.

WHAT IT DOES
Each B vitamin is associated with numerous functions and sometimes works best with other B vitamins. Several of the Bs (B_6, B_{12} and folic acid) are important for reducing the risk of heart disease, which is why B-complex supplements are now so popular. Niacin can reduce high cholesterol levels. Folic acid is also key in reducing spinal cord birth defects and is, therefore, a critical ingredient in prenatal vitamins. (See "ConsumerTips™ for buying and using," page 56.)

QUALITY CONCERNS
After discovering problems with the B-vitamin content of numerous multivitamins in its earlier research on supplements, ConsumerLab.com became concerned about B-vitamin amounts in general (see "Multivitamins & minerals," pages 33 to 49). For example, one prenatal multivitamin had only three-quarters of its claimed folic acid and five multivitamins had niacin levels above the established tolerable upper intake levels (ULs) for tolerable intake from the Institute of Medicine of

the National Academies. Too much niacin increases the likelihood of skin flushing, tingling, and pain with continuous use. Unfortunately, the U.S. Food and Drug Administration (FDA), which regulates labeling, has yet to require that products include information about ULs on labels. (See DRIs reviewed, page 57.)

ConsumerLab.com also was concerned about proper disintegration.

PRODUCT TESTING

ConsumerLab.com purchased 21 dietary supplements claiming to contain single B-vitamins or B-vitamin complexes and tested them for their levels of 7 of the 8 B vitamins: thiamin, riboflavin, total B_3 (niacin and niacinamide), total B_5 (pantothenic acid), total B_6 (pyridoxine and derivatives), folic acid, and total B_{12}. Their ability to break down in solution was evaluated as well. (Chewable and time-release products weren't tested for disintegration.) Biotin wasn't evaluated because no suitable analytical standard exists. (See "ConsumerLab.com's testing methods and standards," page 169.)

TEST FINDINGS

Of the 21 supplements that ConsumerLab.com tested, 14 were single B-vitamin products and 7 were B-vitamin complexes (multiple B vitamins).

ConsumerLab.com found that nine product labels recommended doses that exceeded the ULs for adults. (For amounts above the UL, the risk of adverse reactions increases with regular use.) In fact, all three niacin-only products exceeded the UL, and so did six B-complex products (one of which also exceeded the UL for pyridoxine). The adult UL for niacin is 35 mg/day; for pyridoxine, 100 mg/day (see "ConsumerTips™ for buying and using," page 56). The three niacin-only products recommended daily doses ranging from 400 to 510 mg; the six B-complex products, daily doses ranging from 40 to 150 mg of niacin. (One also recommended 150 mg/day of pyridoxine.)

Although the doses in these products were as much as 10 times higher than the ULs, the products may be appropriate for treating or preventing certain diseases, such as cardiovascular disease, when used under the supervision of a health care professional. Some products were extended-release pills; others contained a slow-release form of niacin (inositol hexanicotinate). Both extended-release and slow-release pills are less likely than regular-release pills to cause skin flushing, which can occur with doses exceeding 50 mg. But the timed-release pills are still known to have serious toxic effects at doses higher than 50 mg.

One of the seven B-complex products was low in thiamin, riboflavin, niacin, and pyridoxine, containing just 76% to 88% of claimed amounts. Products providing less than the claimed amounts may have reduced potency. All 14 of the single B-vitamin products contained the amounts claimed, and all 21 of the products disintegrated properly for absorption.

QUALITY PRODUCTS

Listed alphabetically by name on pages 58 to 63 are the products that passed ConsumerLab.com's independent testing of vitamin B dietary supplements (see B-vitamin and B-complex approved-quality products).

CONSUMERTIPS™ FOR BUYING AND USING

ConsumerLab.com has prepared numerous important tips about dosing, selecting, and buying B vitamin supplements. This information — along with our list of approved-quality brands — provides a valuable guide for choosing appropriate products.

The information in the "The B's" below will help you determine which amounts are appropriate for your gender and life stage. Remember that 1,000 mcg (micrograms) equals 1 mg (milligram) and that 1,000 mg equals 1 gram. (See DRIs reviewed.)

THE B'S

THIAMIN (B₁)

Also spelled thiamine, thiamin (B_1) assists the nervous system. Good food sources include yeast, peas, beans, and grains. If these foods are regularly included in the diet, supplementation is usually unnecessary.

Recommended daily intake: The RDA is 0.5 mg for children ages 1 to 3, 0.6 mg for children ages 4 to 8, and 0.9 mg for children ages 9 to 13. For males ages 14 and older, the RDA is 1.2 mg. For females ages 14 to 18, it's 1.0 mg, and it increases to 1.1 mg for teens ages 19 and older. However, the RDA for pregnant or breast-feeding women is 1.4 mg.

Upper limit: No UL has been established for thiamin.

DRIs reviewed

To ensure that you're getting enough B vitamins to meet basic nutrient requirements and to avoid deficiencies, refer to the recommended daily intakes for each (see "The B's," pages 56 to 69). These values, known as Dietary Reference Intakes (DRIs), have been established by the Institute of Medicine of the National Academies. DRIs come in two types. One type is the Recommended Dietary Allowance (RDA), which is the average daily dietary intake that's sufficient to meet the nutrient requirements of most healthy individuals of a particular gender and life stage. The other type is the Adequate Intake (AI), which is an approximation used when there isn't enough information to develop an RDA. Although the Food and Drug Administration requires supplement labels for certain vitamins and minerals to show the percentage of the Daily Value (% DV) that that supplement accounts for, the percentage given may not reflect the latest RDA or AI. The current DV figures are based on recommended intakes established before 1968, and several have since changed.

If you're buying B vitamins to reduce the risk of heart disease or to treat a medical condition, such as a high cholesterol level, you may need a higher dose than the DRI (see "The B's," page 56 to 69). In any case, be aware that you can get too much of a vitamin. The UL is the highest level of daily nutrient intake unlikely to have adverse health effects. As your intake increases above the UL, your risk of adverse reactions increases. Like the RDAs and AIs, the ULs vary according to gender and life stage. Individuals are advised not to regularly exceed the UL without medical recommendation and supervision. Be aware, too, that products aren't required to indicate that their ingredients exceed the ULs and that many products do exceed those amounts.

RIBOFLAVIN (B$_2$)

Riboflavin (B$_2$) helps maintain vision and skin. Good sources include vegetables and nuts. Supplementation may be needed in children and the elderly.

Recommended daily intake: The RDA is 0.5 mg for children ages 1 to 3, 0.6 mg for children ages 4 to 8, and 0.9 mg for children ages 9 to 13. For males ages 14 and older, the RDA is 1.3 mg. For females ages 14 to 18, it's 1.0 mg, and it increases to 1.1 mg for adults ages 19 and older. The RDA for pregnant women is 1.4 mg and for breast-feeding women

B-vitamin and B-complex approved-quality products

Some products may contain additional ingredients not shown here (see *Ingredients in B-vitamin products,* pages 68 to 69).
Labeled amount of B vitamins (mg/pill unless noted)

Product†	B₁ (Thiamin)	B₂ (Riboflavin)	B₃ (Niacin)
B complexes			
Nature Made® Balanced B-150 B-Complex Supplement Time Released (tablet)1,2 ‡	150	150	150
Dist: Nature Made Nutritional Products			
Nature's Bounty B Complex Vitamins Dietary Supplement (tablet) 1	5	5	40
Mf: Nature's Bounty, Inc.			
Nutrilite Natural B Complex Dietary Supplement (tablet) (Suggested daily serving is 3 tablets.)	1.2	1.2	6.67
Dist: Access Business Group International LLC (formally Amway)			
Puritan's Pride® Inspired by Nature™ Vitamin B-50 B-Complex Vitamin Dietary Supplement (tablet) 1	50	50	50
Mf: Puritan's Pride, Inc.			
Stresstabs® High Potency B-Complex with Antioxidants C & E, & Folic Acid + Zinc Dietary Supplement (tablet) 1	10 .	10	100
Dist: Inverness Medical, Inc			
Vitamin World® Naturally Inspired™ B-100® Ultra B-Complex Dietary Supplement (tablet) 1	100	100	100
Mf: Vitamin World, Inc.			

B₅ (Pantothenic Acid)	B₆ (Pyridoxine)	B₁₂ (Cyanocobalamin; mcg/pill)	Biotin	Folic Acid (mcg/pill)
150	150	150 mcg	150	400 mcg
4.6	1	1 mcg	N/A	N/A
5	1.2	2 mcg	N/A	133.3 mcg
50	50	50 mcg	50	100 mcg
20	5	12 mcg	45	400 mcg
100	100	100 mcg	100	400 mcg

(continued)

Product†	B₁ (Thiamin)	B₂ (Riboflavin)	B₃ (Niacin)

Single B vitamins

B₁ (Thiamin)
TwinLab® B-1 Caps Dietary
Supplement (100 mg/caplet)

	100	N/A	N/A

Mf: Twin Laboratories Inc.

B₃ (Niacin)

Nature's Bounty® Flush Free Niacin Inositol Hexanicotinate 500 mg Dietary Supplement (400 mg/capsule) 1	N/A	N/A	400

Mf: Nature's Bounty, Inc.

Slo Niacin® Polygel® Controlled-release Niacin Dietary Supplement (500 mg/tablet) 1	N/A	N/A	500

Dist: Upsher-Smith Laboratories, Inc.

Thorne Research NiaSafe-600® (510 mg niacin/capsule) 1	N/A	N/A	510

Mf: Thorne Research, Inc. (Julian Whittaker)

B₆ (Pyridoxine)

Marquee Vitamin B-6 Dietary Supplement (100 mg/tablet)	N/A	N/A	N/A

Dist: Fleming Companies, Inc.

Mason Natural® Vitamin B-6 N/A N/A Dietary Supplement (100 mg/tablet)	N/A	N/A	N/A

Mfd. for Mason Vitamins, Inc.

Medicine Shoppe® Vitamin B6 Dietary Supplement (50 mg/tablet)	N/A	N/A	N/A

Dist: Medicine Shoppe International, Inc.

Perfect Choice® Sparks Energy B-6 Vitamin Dietary Supplement (100 mg/tablet)	N/A	N/A	N/A

B$_5$ (Pantothenic Acid)	B$_6$ (Pyridoxine)	B$_{12}$ (Cyanocobalamin; mcg/pill)	Biotin	Folic Acid (mcg/pill)
N/A	N/A	N/A	N/A	N/A
N/A	N/A	N/A	N/A	N/A
N/A	N/A	N/A	N/A	N/A
N/A	N/A	N/A	N/A	N/A
N/A	100	N/A	N/A	N/A
N/A	100	N/A	N/A	N/A
N/A	50	N/A	N/A	N/A
N/A	100	N/A	N/A	N/A

(continued)

B vitamins

Product†	B$_1$ (Thiamin)	B$_2$ (Riboflavin)	B$_3$ (Niacin)
Dist: Inter-American Products, Inc.			
B$_{12}$ (Cobalamin)			
Nature's Valley™ Vitamin B-12 500 mcg Dietary Supplement For Healthy Blood Cells and Nervous System (500 mcg/tablet)	N/A	N/A	N/A
Dist: American Procurement & Logistics Company			
Puritan's Pride® Inspired by Nature™ Vitamin B-12 500 mcg Dietary Supplement (500 mcg/tablet)	N/A	N/A	N/A
Mf: Puritan's Pride, Inc.			
Sav-on™ Natural Time Release Dietary Supplement Vitamin B-12 (1,000 mcg/tablet)	N/A	N/A	N/A
Dist: American Procurement & Logistics Company			
Target Brand Vitamin B12 Dietary Supplement (100 mcg/tablet)	N/A	N/A	N/A
Dist: Target Corporation			
Folic Acid			
Naturvite Natural Vitamins Folic Acid 400 mcg Dietary Supplement (400 mcg/tablet)	N/A	N/A	N/A
Mfd. for Naturvite Natural Vitamins			
Super G Natural Folic Acid 400 mcg Dietary Supplement (400 mcg/tablet)	N/A	N/A	N/A
Dist: Super G, Inc.			

† See "Ingredients in B-vitamin products," pages 68 to 69.
‡ See "More Brand Information," page 191.
1 Exceeds tolerable upper intake level (UL) for niacin; adverse reactions may occur.
2 Exceeds UL for pyridoxine; adverse reactions may occur.
N/A: Not applicable

B$_5$ (Pantothenic Acid)	B$_6$ (Pyridoxine)	B$_{12}$ (Cyanocobalamin; mcg/pill)	Biotin	Folic Acid (mcg/pill)
N/A	N/A	500 mcg	N/A	N/A
N/A	N/A	500 mcg	N/A	N/A
N/A	N/A	1,000 mcg	N/A	N/A
N/A	N/A	100 mcg	N/A	N/A
N/A	N/A	N/A	N/A	400 mcg
N/A	N/A	N/A	N/A	400 mcg

1.6 mg. Much higher amounts (400 mg/day) have been suggested for the prevention of migraines.

Upper limit: No UL has been established for riboflavin.

NIACIN (B₃)

Also known as nicotinic acid, niacin (B_3) helps release energy from carbohydrates and can help lower cholesterol levels, thus reducing the death rate from cardiovascular disease. Niacinamide (or nicotinamide) is another form of niacin that may help prevent diabetes in children at risk for developing it. A third form is called inositol hexanicotinate (or hexaniacinate), and it may help reduce leg cramping caused by atherosclerosis. Good food sources of niacin include enriched white flour, peanuts, fish, and meat.

Recommended daily intake: The RDA is 6 mg for children ages 1 to 3, 8 mg for children ages 4 to 8, and 12 mg for children ages 9 to 13. For males ages 14 and older, the RDA is 16 mg. For females ages 14 and older, it's 14 mg. The RDA for pregnant women is 18 mg and for breast-feeding women 17 mg. Dosages used for treating diseases range from 1,000 to 4,000 mg/day (1 to 4 grams/day), levels that are significantly higher than the RDAs and ULs. Also, be aware that the amount of niacin in inositol hexanicotinate is about 85%, meaning that if a product contains 600 mg of inositol hexanicotinate, it has about 500 mg of niacin.

Upper limit: Daily doses that exceed 50 mg have been associated with skin flushing, including reddening, burning, tingling, itching, and pain. Taking niacin with food and starting with a lower dose, then gradually increasing the amount, may reduce this adverse effect. Slow-release niacin and products made from nicotinamide (or niacinamide) and inositol hexanicotinate are also less likely to cause flushing. However, liver toxicity may occur with daily doses of niacin that exceed 1,500 mg (1.5 grams) or daily doses of nicotinamide that exceed 3,000 mg (3 grams). Toxic reactions are most common in people taking slow-release niacin. The UL for niacin, which applies only to amounts consumed from supplements and fortified foods, is 10 mg for children ages 1 to 3, 15 mg for children ages 4 to 8, 20 mg for children ages 9 to 13, 30 mg for teens ages 14 to 18, and 35 mg for adults ages 19 and older.

Caution: Niacinamide may increase blood levels of anticonvulsants.

PANTOTHENIC ACID

Sometimes called vitamin B$_5$, pantothenic acid is involved in energy production as well as hormone and neurotransmitter synthesis. Although deficiency is rare, it's seen in alcoholics. Especially good sources of pantothenic acid include liver, yeast, and salmon.

Recommended daily intake: The AI is 2 mg for children ages 1 to 3, 3 mg for children ages 4 to 8, and 4 mg for children ages 9 to 13. For individuals ages 14 and older, the AI is 5 mg. The AI for pregnant women is 6 mg and for women who breast-feeding 7 mg. Daily doses up to 900 mg have been used to reduce high cholesterol levels.

Upper limit: No UL has been established for pantothenic acid.

PYRIDOXINE (B$_6$)

Pyridoxine (B$_6$) is important for metabolism as well as for maintenance of the immune and nervous systems. It may also reduce both nausea from morning sickness and the risk of heart disease. Pyridoxine in amounts that meet the RDAs is easily available from food, however mild deficiency is common, particularly in children and the elderly. Good sources of pyridoxine include avocados, bananas, brewer's yeast, buckwheat flour, lentils, lima beans, soybeans, sunflower seeds, walnuts, and wheat germ.

Recommended daily intake: The RDA is 0.5 mg for children ages 1 to 3, 0.6 mg for children ages 4 to 8, and 1.0 mg for children ages 9 to 13. For males ages 14 to 50, the RDA is 1.3 mg; for males older than age 51, 1.7 mg. For females ages 14 to 18, the RDA is 1.2 mg; for females ages 19 to 50, 1.3 mg; and for females older than age 51, 1.5 mg. The RDA for pregnant women is 1.9 mg and for breast-feeding women 2.0 mg. To help reduce the risk of heart disease, about 5 mg/day is recommended; to help reduce the nausea of morning sickness, about 30 mg/day is recommended.

Upper limit: Too much pyridoxine (more than 1 gram/day) can cause nerve damage and skin lesions. The UL is 30 mg for children ages 1 to 3, 40 mg for children ages 4 to 8, 60 mg for children ages 9 to 13, 80 mg for teens ages 14 to 18, and 100 mg for adults ages 19 and older.

FOLIC ACID

Also known as folate, folacin, and B$_9$, folic acid reduces the risk of the birth defect spina bifida (a leading cause of childhood paralysis). It may also reduce the risk of heart disease and childhood leukemia. Good sources include dark green leafy vegetables and oranges. Most people can get sufficient folic acid from their diet, but supplements are generally recommended for women who may soon become pregnant and for pregnant women.

Recommended daily intake: The RDAs are based on food sources, but the folic acid in supplements and fortified foods is absorbed twice as easily. Consequently, if you're relying on supplements or fortified foods to reach the RDA, you need only half the amount listed in the following RDAs: 150 mcg for children ages 1 to 3, 200 mcg for children ages 4 to 8, and 300 mcg for children ages 9 to 13. For individuals ages 14 and older, the RDA is 400 mcg. For pregnant women, it's 600 mcg and for breast-feeding women 500 mcg. Because folic acid is critical to developing fetuses during the first few weeks after conception, all women capable of becoming pregnant should consume 400 mcg from supplements or fortified foods in addition to eating a varied diet rich in folic acid.

Upper limit: Prolonged intake of excess folic acid can cause kidney damage and can complicate the diagnosis of vitamin B_{12} deficiency (primarily seen in older adults). The UL for folic acid, which applies only to the amount consumed from supplements and fortified foods, is 300 mcg for children ages 1 to 3, 400 mcg for children ages 4 to 8, 600 mcg for children ages 9 to 13, and 800 mcg for teens ages 14 to 18. For adults ages 19 and older, the UL is 1,000 mcg.

CYANOCOBALAMIN (B_{12})

A cyanocobalamin, or vitamin B_{12}, deficiency can cause anemia, irreversible nerve damage, and low sperm count. When used with vitamin B_6, it can reduce the risk of heart disease. Vitamin B_{12} is abundant in meats; it's also plentiful in poultry and fish. A healthful diet should meet the vitamin B_{12} RDAs, but strict vegetarians, alcohol and drug abusers, people recovering from surgery or burns, or those with bowel or pancreatic cancer may need to take a supplement. Deficiency is also common in people with low stomach acidity (common in older individuals) because the vitamin is difficult to absorb from foods. Consequently, people older than age 50 may want to consider taking a supplement and consuming fortified foods.

Recommended daily intake: The RDA is 0.9 mcg for children ages 1 to 3, 1.2 mcg for children ages 4 to 8, and 1.8 mcg for children ages 9 to 13. For individuals older than age 14, the RDA is 2.4 mcg. For pregnant women, it's 2.6 mcg and for breast-feeding women 2.8 mcg. Higher doses of vitamin B_{12} (about 400 mcg/day) are used to help prevent heart disease.

Upper limit: No UL has been established for vitamin B_{12}.

BIOTIN

Biotin is needed for metabolizing other nutrients. Deficiency is rare under normal circumstances because bacteria in the gut can produce biotin. Good sources of the nutrient include organ meats, oatmeal, egg yolk, mushrooms, bananas, peanuts, and brewer's yeast. Long-term use of antibiotics or anticonvulsants can cause a biotin deficiency.

Recommended daily intake: The AI for biotin is 8 mcg for children ages 1 to 3, 12 mcg for children ages 4 to 8, and 20 mcg for children ages 9 to 13. For teens ages 14 to 18, the AI is 25 mcg; for adults ages 19 and older, it's 30 mcg. The AI increases to 35 mcg for breast-feeding women.

Upper limit: No UL has been established for biotin.

CAUTIONS AND CONCERNS

B vitamins are safe when taken in appropriate amounts, but aware that B vitamins shouldn't be taken in excess. If you must exceed the ULs, do so under a physician's supervision, and be alert to potential adverse effects.

Remember, too, certain B vitamins can interact with drugs and other supplements.

Ingredients in B-vitamin products

Suggested daily serving is 1 pill, unless otherwise specified.

B complexes

Nature Made Balanced B-150 B-Complex Supplement Time Released
Thiamin 150 mg; Riboflavin 150 mg; Niacin 150 mg; Vitamin B_6 150 mg; Folate 400 mcg; Vitamin B_{12} 150 mcg; Biotin 150 mcg; Pantothenic Acid 150 mg

Nature's Bounty B Complex Vitamins Dietary Supplement
Thiamin (Vitamin B_1) (as Thiamine Hydrochloride) 5 mg; Riboflavin (Vitamin B_2) 5 mg; Niacin (as Niacinamide) 40 mg; Vitamin B_6 (as Pyridoxine Hydrochloride) 1 mg; Vitamin B_{12} (as Cyanocobalamin) 1 mcg; Pantothenic Acid (as d-Calcium Pantothenate) 4.6 mg; Inositol 10 mg; Choline Bitartrate 20 mg; Desiccated Liver Powder 100 mg; Brewer's Yeast 50 mg

Nutrilite Natural B Complex Dietary Supplement
(Suggested daily serving is 3 tablets; ingredient levels are shown for a single tablet.)
Thiamin 1.2 mg; Riboflavin 1.2 mg; Niacin 6.6.7 mg; Vitamin B_6 1.2 mg; Folic Acid 133.33 mcg; Vitamin B_{12} 2 mcg; Pantothenic Acid 5 mg; Inositol 3.6 mg; Para-Aminobenzoic Acid 3 mg

Puritan's Pride® Inspired by Nature™ Vitamin B-50 B-Complex Vitamin Dietary Supplement
Thiamin (Vitamin B_1 as Thiamin Mononitrate) 50 mg; Riboflavin (Vitamin B_2) 50 mg; Niacin (as Niacinamide) 50 mg; Vitamin B_6 (as Pyridoxine Hydrochloride) 50 mg; Folic Acid 100 mcg; Vitamin B_{12} (as Cyanocobalamin) 50 mcg; Biotin (as d-Biotin) 50 mcg; Pantothenic Acid (as d-Calcium Pantothenate) 50 mg; PABA (Para-Aminobenzoic Acid) 50 mg; Inositol 50 mg; Choline Bitartrate 50 mg; Proprietary Blend (Alfalfa, Watercress, Parsley, Lecithin; Rice Bran) 2.5 mg

Stresstabs® High Potency B-Complex with Antioxidants C & E, & Folic Acid + Zinc Dietary Supplemen
Vitamin C (as Ascorbic Acid) 500 mg; Vitamin E (as dl-Alpha Tocopheryl Acetate) 30 I.U.; Thiamin (as Thiamin Mononitrate) 10 mg; Riboflavin 10 mg; Niacinamide 100 mg; Vitamin B6 (as Pyridoxine Hydrochloride) 5 mg; Folic Acid 400 mcg; Vitamin B_{12} (as Cyanocobalamin) 12 mcg; Biotin 45 mcg; Pantothenic Acid (as d-Calcium Pantothenate) 20 mg; Zinc (as Zinc Oxide) 23.9 mg; Copper (as Cupric Oxide) 3 mg

Vitamin World® Naturally Inspired™ B-100® Ultra B-Complex Dietary Supplement
Thiamin (Vitamin B_1) (as Thiamine Mononitrate) 100 mg; Riboflavin (Vitamin B_2) 100 mg; Niacin (as Niacinamide) 100 mg; Vitamin B6 (as Pyridoxine Hydrochloride) 100 mg; Folic Acid 400 mcg; Vitamin B_{12} (as Cyanocobalamin) 100 mcg; Biotin (as d-Biotin) 100 mcg; Pantothenic Acid (as d-Calcium Pantothenate) 100 mg; Inositol 100 mg; PABA (Para-Aminobenzoic Acid) 100 mg; Choline Bitartrate 100 mg; Proprietary Blend (Parsley Leaves Powder, Rice Bran Defatted Powder, Watercress Leaves Powder, Alfalfa Leaves Powder, Lecithin Granules)

B₁ (Thiamin)

TwinLab® B1 Caps Dietary Supplement
Thiamin (from Thiamin Mononitrate) 100 mg

Niacin (B₃)

Nature's Bounty® Flush Free Niacin Inositol Hexanicotinate 500 mg Dietary Supplement
Niacin (as Inositol Hexanicotinate) 400 mg; Inositol (as Inositol Hexanicotinate) 100 mg

Slo Niacin® polygel® controlled-release niacin Dietary Supplement 500 mg
Niacin, USP (nicotinic acid) 500 mg

Thorne Research NiaSafe-600®
Niacin (from 600 mg Inositol Hexanicotinate*) 510 mg (*Doesn't cause flushing in most people.)

B₆ (Pyridoxine)

Marquee Vitamin B6 Dietary Supplement
Vitamin B₆ 100 mg

Mason natural® Vitamin B6 100 mg Dietary Supplement
Vitamin B₆ (Pyridoxine Hydrochloride) 100 mg; Calcium (Dicalcium Phosphate) 62 mg

Medicine Shoppe® Vitamin B6 50 mg (Pyridoxine Hydrochloride) Dietary Supplement
Vitamin B₆ 50 mg

Perfect Choice® Sparks Energy B6 Vitamin Dietary Supplement
Vitamin B₆ 100 mg

B₁₂ (Colbalamin)

Nature's Valley™ Vitamin B12 500 mcg Dietary Supplement For Healthy Blood Cells and Nervous System
Vitamin B₁₂ 500 mcg

Puritan's Pride® Inspired by Nature™ Vitamin B12 500 mcg Dietary Supplement
Vitamin B₁₂ (as cyanocobalamin) 500 mcg

Sav-on™ Natural Time release Dietary Supplement Vitamin B12 1000 mcg
Vitamin B₁₂ 1000 mcg

Target Brand Vitamin B12 Dietary Supplement
Vitamin B₁₂ 100 mcg

Folic Acid

Naturvite Natural Vitamins Folic Acid 400 mcg Dietary Supplement
Folic Acid 400 mcg; Calcium (as Dicalcium Phosphate) 70 mg

Super G Natural Folic Acid 400 mcg Dietary Supplement
Folate 400 mcg

Vitamin C

WHAT IT IS

Vitamin C (ascorbic acid or dehydroascorbic acid) is an essential water-soluble vitamin that the human body can't manufacture. It must, therefore, come from foods or supplements. Fruits and vegetables are the richest food sources of vitamin C. Dietary supplements are typically sold as ascorbic acid, calcium ascorbate (Ester-C®), sodium ascorbate, or a combination of these forms. Vitamin C supplements also commonly contain rose hips, a high-quality vitamin C source. Rose hips are the pear-shaped fruit of the rose, without the flower's petals. Vitamin C is available in buffered and slow-release forms to reduce digestive problems, which typically occur with very high doses.

WHAT IT DOES

Vitamin C helps the body produce collagen, a basic component of connective tissue. Collagen is an important structural element in blood vessel walls, gums, and bones, making it particularly important to anyone recovering from wounds or surgery. Vitamin C also acts as an antioxidant, scavenging potentially harmful molecules called free radicals. Although not firmly established by clinical trials, this antioxidant activity may help boost immune function and protect against cancer, cataracts, age-related macular degeneration of the retina, and other chronic diseases. Vitamin C intake may be particularly helpful to smokers, who may suffer from oxidative stress and cell damage, which can deplete the body's store of vitamin C. Vitamin C also enhances iron absorption from supplements and plant foods. A recent study, however, suggests that vitamin C and other antioxidants may reduce the effectiveness of cholesterol-lowering drugs.

70

Good sources of vitamin C include many vegetables, such as broccoli and brussels sprouts, as well citrus and other fruits. A healthful diet should provide the Recommended Dietary Allowance (RDA).

QUALITY CONCERNS

Regulations from the U.S. Food and Drug Administration (FDA) require that any vitamin C sold as a dietary supplement in the United States contain at least 100% of its labeled amount. The United States Pharmacopeia (USP) requires that products contain 90% to 110% of the claimed amount and that they meet certain specifications for disintegration and purity. Unfortunately, the FDA doesn't test for quality before sales, and products stating that they meet the USP standards don't always do so. Therefore, ConsumerLab.com tested several leading vitamin C dietary supplements to determine whether they contained 100% of the labeled amounts of vitamin C and whether they disintegrated properly.

PRODUCT TESTING

ConsumerLab.com purchased 26 brands of vitamin C products, including 5 products for children. Of these, 7 claimed USP quality on their labels. All were tested for their levels of vitamin C and their ability to break down in solution. Chewable and time-release products weren't tested for disintegration. (See "ConsumerLab.com's testing methods and standards," page 169.)

TEST FINDINGS

Of the 26 brands of vitamin C products that ConsumerLab.com tested, 4 products, or 15%, didn't pass testing. Of these, 1 product failed to break down properly, and 3 products didn't contain enough vitamin C. Of these 3, 1 indicated it was USP quality, but analysis showed it had only 88% of the labeled amount. The other 2 failing products, 1 of which was a children's vitamin, had 94% and 95% of their claimed amounts of vitamin C.

The failure rate was about the same for USP and non-USP labeled products. Of the passing products, those with the USP label tended to have slightly less than 100% of the stated amount of vitamin C. The opposite was true of the non-USP labeled products: they tended to have somewhat more than 100% of the stated amount.

QUALITY PRODUCTS

Listed alphabetically by name on pages 74 to 75 are the products that passed ConsumerLab.com's independent testing to vitamin C dietary supplements (see Vitamin C approved-quality products).

CONSUMERTIPS™ FOR BUYING AND USING

ConsumerLab.com has prepared numerous important tips about dosing, selecting, and buying vitamin C supplements. This information—along with our list of approved-quality brands—provides a valuable guide for choosing appropriate products.

Both natural and synthetic vitamin C are equally recognized and used by the body, so don't pay more for an all-natural rose-hips product. In fact, some products stating "with rose hips" but not indicating the amount may contain far more synthetic vitamin C (or another natural source) than rose hips. Even binders and fillers, such as cellulose, are often present in greater amounts than rose hips. (Hint: A product's ingredient list gives a clue to the amount of rose hips present. Ingredients on that list must appear in the order of amount, from greatest to least. If rose hips appear last, there isn't much in the product.) In fact, one company we contacted said only 10% of their product's vitamin C came from rose hips.

The following information about recommended intakes will help you determine which amounts are appropriate for your gender and life stage. Remember that 1,000 mcg (micrograms) equals 1 mg (milligram) and that 1,000 mg equals 1 gram. (See Understanding Recommended Dietary Allowances, Adequate Intakes, Tolerable Upper Intake Levels, page 46.)

Recommended daily intake: In April 2000, the RDA for vitamin C was increased to provide antioxidant protection. The RDA is 90 mg for adult males and 75 mg for adult females. An additional 35 mg is recommended for smokers. For pregnant women ages 18 and younger, the RDA is 80 mg and for pregnant women older than age 18, it's 85 mg.

For breast-feeding women ages 18 years and younger, the RDA is 115 mg and for breast-feeding women older than age 18, it's 120 mg.

The RDAs for children are 15 mg for ages 1 to 3, 25 mg for ages 4 to 8, and 45 mg for ages 9 to 13. For males ages 14 to 18, the RDA is 75 mg. For females ages 14 to 18, it's 65 mg.

The RDAs are easily achievable with healthful diets high in vitamin-C-rich fruits and vegetables and are also more than adequate for normal collagen production. However, some health care professionals recommend higher daily doses of vitamin C, such as 500 to 1,500 mg for adults, to stimulate the immune system.

Upper limit: When giving vitamin C to children, remember that the established tolerable upper level intake (UL) is 400 mg for children ages 1 to 3; 650 mg for children ages 4 to 8, 1,200 mg for children ages 9 to 13; 1,800 mg for teens ages 14 to 18. For individuals ages 19 and older, the UL is 2,000 mg. Don't exceed these levels without medical supervision.

CAUTIONS AND CONCERNS

Vitamin C is safe when taken in moderate amounts, but be aware that too much vitamin C from supplements can cause diarrhea and other gastric disturbances, and may contribute to kidney and bladder stones. What's more, a recent test-tube study showed that vitamin C may cause the production of DNA-damaging genotoxins and may promote the development of cancer, supporting the notion that taking excess vitamin C may not reduce cancer risk. Thus, caution is appropriate when taking excess vitamin C: avoid consuming more than 2,000 mg a day.

Vitamin C may interfere with the absorption of tricyclic antidepressants and anticoagulants. Also, excess vitamin C from supplements can interfere with several diagnostic tests for cholesterol and blood sugar levels, and blood in the stool.

Vitamin C approved-quality products

Product name concentration/pill and form)	Manufacturer (Mf) or distributor (Dist)
Bio C Plus (250 mg, as ascorbic acid)* ‡	Mf: Nutrilite (Access Business Group International LLC)
CVS C vitamin (500 mg, USP, as ascorbic acid)	Dist: CVS
Ester-C® (250 mg, as calcium ascorbate)	Mf: Natrol, Inc.
Kirkland Signature Natural Vitamin C (1,000 mg with Rose Hips, USP, as ascorbic acid)	Dist: CWC, Inc.
Natural Wealth Natural C-500 (500 mg with Rose Hips, USP, as ascorbic acid)	Mf: Natural Wealth
Nature Made Vitamin C (1000 mg Supplement, as ascorbic acid)‡	Dist: Nature Made Nutritional Products
Nature's Bounty Natural Vitamin C-1000 (1,000 mg, USP, as ascorbic acid)	Mf: Nature's Bounty, Inc.
Nature's Way Vitamin C (1000 mg with rose hips, as ascorbic acid)	Dist: Nature's Way Products, Inc.
One A Day Cold Season (500 mg, as ascorbic acid)	Dist: Bayer
Schiff Vitamin C with Rose Hips (500 mg, as ascorbic acid)	Dist: Schiff Products, Inc.
Super Ester-C® with Bioflavonoids, (500 mg, as calcium ascorbate)	Mf: Whole Foods Market, Inc.
Spring Valley Vitamin C (500 mg, as ascorbic acid)	Mf: Leiner Health Products, Inc.
Sunkist Vitamin C Citrus Complex Chewable (500 mg, as sodium ascorbate and ascorbic acid)	Dist: Novartis Consumer Health, Inc.
Vita-C (100 mg Chewable Vitamin C, as ascorbic acid)	Dist: Shaklee Corp.
Vitamin C-500 (500 mg, as ascorbic acid)	Mf: Puritans Pride, Inc.
Windmill Natural Rose Hips with Vitamin C (500 mg, as ascorbic acid)	Dist: Windmill Vitamin Co., Inc.
Walgreens Vitamin C with Rose Hips (500 mg USP, as ascorbic acid)	Dist: Walgreens
Your Life Natural Vitamin C (500 mg with Rose Hips, USP, as ascorbic acid)	Dist: Your Life

Product name concentration/pill and form)	Manufacturer (Mf) or distributor (Dist)
Children's Brands	
Centrum Kids Chewable Vitamins with Extra C, Shamu and his Crew (250 mg, as ascorbic acid and sodium ascorbate)‡	Dist: Whitehall-Robins Healthcare
CTW Sesame Street Extra C Multi-Vitamin Supplement (80 mg, as ascorbic acid)	Dist: McNeil Consumer Healthcare/ Johnson and Johnson
Naturally Kid's JuiCee (60 mg, as calcium ascorbate)	Dist: Naturally Vitamins
Thompson Vitamin C Children's Chewable (100 mg Natural Orange Flavor, as sodium ascorbate and ascorbic acid)	Dist: Thompson Nutritional Products

* Tested through ConsumerLab.com's Ad Hoc Testing Program (Product was tested at the manufacturer's request after the initial review was completed and released.)

‡ See "More Brand Information," page 191.

Vitamin E

WHAT IT IS

Vitamin E is a family of related molecules called tocopherols. Of the several types of tocopherols that are available, alpha-tocopherol is the most biologically active. Alpha-tocopherol can exist in eight different forms, but the body can only use half of these forms.

Natural vitamin E, alpha-tocopherol, may also contain other types of tocopherols, such as beta-tocopherol, delta-tocopherol, and gamma-tocopherol. Some manufacturers use the term "mixed" tocopherols when referring to these different types. Investigations are underway to determine whether gamma-tocopherol, which is more abundant in the diet than alpha-tocopherol, may be important for some of the beneficial effects associated with dietary vitamin E. Synthetic vitamin E (sometimes referred to as dl-alpha-tocopherol) contains both active and inactive forms of alpha-tocopherol.

WHAT IT DOES

Vitamin E (tocopherol) is an antioxidant that helps maintain cell integrity. Only a relatively small amount of vitamin E is required to meet normal daily requirements. Fortunately, this amount is easily obtained from foods, including sunflower oil, safflower oil, canola oil, olive oil, whole grains, nuts, fruits, and the fatty parts of meats. Consequently, vitamin E deficiency is rare in the United States. However, research using high doses of vitamin E suggests that the vitamin may be beneficial in preventing prostate and other cancers, as well as in treating or preventing tardive dyskinesia, restless leg syndrome, acute anterior uveitis (inflammation of eye tissues), preeclampsia, Alzheimer's disease, rheumatoid arthritis, and diabetes, among other conditions. Although long-touted for preventing cardiovascular disease, this use hasn't been well demonstrated. In fact, a recent study suggests that vitamin E and other antioxidants may reduce the effectiveness of cholesterol-lowering drugs.

QUALITY CONCERNS

Because no government agency is responsible for routinely testing vitamin E supplements for their contents or quality, ConsumerLab.com independently evaluated several of the leading vitamin E products to determine whether they contained the types and amounts of vitamin E stated on their labels.

PRODUCT TESTING

ConsumerLab.com purchased 28 different vitamin E products: 19 labeled as natural vitamin E, 8 capsules labeled as synthetic vitamin E, and 1 cream labeled as synthetic vitamin E. The products were tested to determine whether they correctly identified the vitamin E type and amount. (See "ConsumerLab.com's testing methods and standards," page 169.)

TEST FINDINGS

Of the 28 products that ConsumerLab.com tested, 3 products failed testing: One synthetic product had no more than 71% of its claimed vitamin E, which was a different chemical form from the one stated on the label. One natural product had no more than 85% of the claimed amount. A third product was labeled as natural but actually contained the synthetic form, albeit in the correct labeled amount; the label's "Supplement Facts" panel indicated that "dl-alpha-tocopherol," which is the synthetic vitamin E, was what the product contained.

QUALITY PRODUCTS

Listed alphabetically by name on pages 78 to 79 are the products that passed ConsumerLab.com's independent testing of vitamin E dietary supplements (see Vitamin E approved-quality products.)

Vitamin E approved-quality products

Product name (labeled type and amount/pill or unit)	Manufacturer (Mf) or distributor (Dist)
Natural Softgel/Capsules/Tab	
Brite-Life® Natural Vitamin E Supplement (400 I.U. softgel)	Dist: Bergen Brunswig Drug Company
Carlson® E-Gems Vitamin E (400 I.U. softgel)	Dist: Carlson Division of J.R. Carlson Laboratories, Inc.
Carlson® Key-E Vitamin E (200 I.U. Chewable Tablets)	Dist: Carlson Division of J.R. Carlson Laboratories, Inc.
Drugstore.com™ Natural Vitamin E d-Alpha Dietary Supplement USP (400 I.U. softgel)	Dist: drugstore.com, Inc.
Kal® Vitamin E-400 Unesterified d-Alpha Tocopherol Fast Acting Dietary Supplement (400 I.U. d-alpha tocopherol softgel)	Mf: Nutraceutical Corp. for Makers of KAL, Inc.
Life Extension™ Vitamin E Capsules, Pure Natural Vitamin E (400 I.U. capsule)	Dist: Life Extension Foundation Buyers Club, Inc.
Natural Factors® E (400 I.U. softgel)	Dist: Natural Factors
Nature's Way® Vitamin E 400 natural d-alpha Dietary Supplement (400 I.U. softgel)	Dist: Nature's Way Products, Inc.
Nutrilite Parselenium E Dietary Supplement (400 I.U. tablet) ‡	Mf: Nutrilite, a Division of Access Business Group International LLC
PharmAssure™ Vitamin E Dietary Supplement, 100% Natural Source (400 I.U. d-alpha tocopherols, softgel)	Dist: PharmAssure, Inc.
Puritan's Pride, Inspired by Nature Natural Vitamin E D-Alpha Tocopheryl, USP Dietary Supplement (400 I.U. d-alpha tocopheryl, softgel)*	Mf: Puritan's Pride, Inc.
Schiff® Natural Vitamin E, d-alpha tocopherol Dietary Supplement (400 I.U. d-alpha tocopherol, softgel)	Dist: Schiff Products, Inc.
Shaklee® Vita-E Plus™ Natural Vitamin E & Selenium with Grapeseed Extract Dietary Supplement (400 I.U. softgel)	Dist: Shaklee Corp.
Solgar Natural Vitamin E 400 I.U. Dietary Supplement (400 I.U. d-alpha tocopherol, softgel)	Dist: Solgar Vitamin and Herb

Product name (labeled type and amount/pill or unit)	Manufacturer (Mf) or distributor (Dist)
Trader Darwin's™ For Survival of the Fittest 100% Natural Vitamin E Dietary Supplement (400 I.U. softgel)	Dist: Trader Joe's
Twinlab® E-400 Caps, 100% Natural, Yeast-Free Dry Vitamin E (400 I.U. capsule)	Mf: Twin Laboratories Inc.
USANA® Optimizers E-Prime™ Vitamin E Supplement (200 I.U. softgel)	Dist: USANA, Inc.
Vitamins.com 100% Natural Vitamin E Mixed Tocopherols (400 I.U. softgel)	Dist: Vitamins.com

Synthetic Softgel/Capsules/Tablets

Kirkland Signature™ High Potency Vitamin E Dietary Supplement (1000 I.U. softgel)	Dist: CWC, Inc.
Kroger® E Vitamin USP Dietary Supplement (400 I.U. softgel)	Dist: The Kroger Co.
Meijer™ Vitamin E Dietary Supplement (400 I.U. softgel)	Dist: Meijer, Inc.
Nature Made® E Vitamin Supplement (400 I.U. softgel) ‡	Dist: Nature Made Nutritional Products
Nature's Bounty Vitamin E (synthetic), USP Dietary Supplement (400 I.U. softgel)*	Mf: Nature's Bounty, Inc.
Shop Rite® Vitamin E Dietary Supplement (400 I.U. softgel)	Dist: Wakefern Food Corp.
VitaSmart® Vitamin E dl-Alpha, Confirmed Release Dietary Supplement (400 I.U. softgel)	Dist: Kmart Corporation
Windmill Vitamin E (200 I.U. softgel)	Dist: Windmill Vitamin Co, Inc.

Creams

Nature's Bounty® Vitamin E-Cream (6,000 I.U. of Vitamin E per jar)	Mf: Nature's Bounty, Inc.

* Tested through ConsumerLab.com's Ad Hoc Testing Program (Product was tested at the manufacturer's request after the initial review was completed and released.)

‡ See "More Brand Information," page 191.

CONSUMERTIPS™ FOR BUYING AND USING

ConsumerLab.com has prepared numerous important tips about dosing, selecting, and buying vitamin E supplements. This information — along with our list of approved-quality brands — provides a valuable guide for choosing appropriate products.

Natural and synthetic vitamin E, in the proper dosages, can be equally active. But, more synthetic vitamin E is required to meet a specific amount of active vitamin E than the natural version. At high doses, however, less synthetic vitamin E is required to cause bleeding problems.

Natural products may not be as they appear. To check, refer to the chemical name on the ingredient label. Natural vitamin E should appear as "d-alpha-tocopherol" or "mixed tocopherols"; dl-alpha-tocopherol is the synthetic version. Acceptable variations include "tocopheryl" instead of "tocopherol," followed by "acetate," "succinate," or "acid succinate."

Recommended daily dosages for basic needs and suggested dosages for preventing and treating certain diseases are wide ranging, which is why some products contain as little as 100 International Units (IUs) of vitamin E per pill and others as much as 1,000 (IUs) per pill. When comparing the costs of vitamin E products, consider the dosage and the number of pills per bottle. (See the next paragraph for conversion information.) Natural vitamin E generally costs more than synthetic vitamin E for equivalent IUs, but this may even out when converting the dosages to milligrams (one IU of natural vitamin E provides 50% more active alpha-tocopherol than one IU of synthetic vitamin E). A cream claiming to contain vitamin E should, at a minimum, state the amount in the product. Many do not. (See Understanding Recommended Dietary Allowances, Adequate Intakes, Tolerable Upper Intake Levels, page 46.)

Recommended daily intake: The Recommended Dietary Allowance (RDA) for vitamin E is based on milligrams of active alpha-tocopherol. Consequently, the amount of vitamin E needed to meet the RDA is different for natural and synthetic versions. However, most supplements are labeled using IUs and not milligrams. Complicating matters a bit, the conversion factors for synthetic and natural vitamin E differ: one IU of synthetic vitamin E equals 0.45 mg of active alpha-tocopherol, whereas one IU of natural vitamin E equals 0.67 mg of active alpha-tocopherol.

Based on these conversion rates, the RDA for vitamin E as active alpha-tocopherol is 6 mg (13 IU synthetic or 9 IU natural) for children ages 1 to 3, 7 mg (16 IU synthetic or 10 IU natural) for children ages 4 to 8, and 11 mg (24 IU synthetic or 16 IU natural) for children ages 9 to 13. For individuals ages 14 and older, the RDA is 15 mg (33 IU synthetic or 22 IU natural). For breast-feeding women, it's 19 mg (42 IU synthetic or 28 IU natural).

It's difficult to consume more than 30 mg of vitamin E per day from food alone, so obtaining higher doses generally requires taking supplements.

Upper limits: Tolerable upper intake levels (ULs) have been established for vitamin E consumed from supplements and fortified foods and represent the highest level of daily intake unlikely to pose a risk of adverse health effects. As intake increases above the UL, the risk of adverse effects may increase, so it's advisable not to regularly exceed the UL without medical recommendation and supervision.

ULs for synthetic vitamin E are lower than those for natural vitamin E. The ULs, therefore, translate approximately to the following IU amounts per day: 200 mg (220 IU synthetic or 300 IU natural) for children ages 1 to 3, 300 mg (330 IU synthetic or 450 IU natural) for children ages 4 to 8, 600 mg (660 IU synthetic or 900 IU natural) for children ages 9 to 13, 800 mg (880 IU synthetic or 1,200 IU natural) for teens ages 14 to 18, and 1,000 mg (1,100 IU synthetic or 1,500 IU natural) for adults ages 19 and older.

CAUTIONS AND CONCERNS

Vitamin E is safe when taken in moderate amounts, but be aware that too much vitamin E may cause bleeding and lead to hemorrhaging. Both the active and inactive forms of alpha-tocopherol found in synthetic vitamin E may contribute to this effect on blood clotting.

If a natural vitamin E product is incorrectly labeled and is actually made from synthetic E, users taking very high doses of vitamin E could find themselves exceeding the upper level without realizing it.

Individuals who are taking an anticoagulant such as coumadin or who are vitamin K deficient should take vitamin E supplements only under a physician's supervision; excessive bleeding is a potential concern for these individuals.

Calcium

WHAT IT IS

Calcium is an essential mineral and is one of the most popular dietary supplements in the United States. Although sufficient calcium can be obtained exclusively from food, especially from dairy products and green leafy vegetables, many people don't get the recommended amount.

Calcium supplements are available in an increasing variety of forms, including tablets, caplets, softgels, syrups, chewable tablets, soft chewable squares, antacids, and calcium-fortified juices. The most common and generally least expensive form of calcium is calcium carbonate (including oyster shell), which is best absorbed when taken with meals, as are most other types of calcium. Calcium citrate malate is an exception: It's taken without food. However, calcium citrate malate as well as calcium lactate and calcium gluconate are bulky compounds, meaning that more pills or larger pills must be taken.

WHAT IT DOES

Calcium is critical for building and maintaining strong bones and teeth, where 99% of the mineral is found in the body. The rest is present in blood, extracellular fluid, muscles, and other tissues, where it plays a role in contraction and vasodilation, muscle contraction, nerve transmission, and glandular secretions.

QUALITY CONCERNS

Like other supplements, neither the U.S. Food and Drug Administration (FDA) nor any other federal or state agency routinely tests calcium products for quality. However, calcium supplements can have certain quality problems.

Labeled Amount: Does the product really contain the labeled amount of calcium? Although calcium is an inexpensive raw material, it can be bulky, making the formulation of calcium supplements complex. If not manufactured properly, products may not contain the labeled amount.

Purity: Does the product contain lead? Many sources of calcium naturally do. In children, infants, and fetuses, even low levels of lead can adversely affect neurobehavioral development and cognitive function. In adults, lead can cause elevated blood pressure and anemia, and it can adversely affect the nervous and reproductive systems. During pregnancy, lead in the mother's body can transfer to the fetus.

ConsumerLab.com purchased many of the leading calcium supplements and calcium-fortified products sold in the United States and independently evaluated them to determine whether they contained the amount of calcium claimed on their labels and whether they were free from harmful levels of lead and other metals.

PRODUCT TESTING

ConsumerLab.com purchased 35 brands of calcium-containing products, several of which also contained other vitamins or minerals, such as magnesium and vitamin D. The brands included 22 nonchewable calcium tablets, softgels, or syrups; 4 chewable antacid tablets; 2 adult chewable tablets or soft chews; 5 children's chewable tablets; and 2 calcium-fortified orange juices. Products were tested for calcium as well as contamination with lead, arsenic, and cadmium. (See "ConsumerLab.com's testing methods and standards," page 169.)

TEST FINDINGS

Of the 35 products that ConsumerLab.com tested, 4 products failed testing — 2 nonchewable tablets, 1 syrup, and 1 caplet. All failed because of low calcium levels, specifically no more than 53% and 91% (nonchewable tablets), 82% (syrup) and 61% (caplet) of the claimed amounts, respectively. Of the 4, 3 didn't carry the USP designation, indicating that the product was produced according to the standards set by the USP. The USP, however, doesn't verify that products bearing its designation meet its standards.

No product failed testing for excessive levels of lead, cadmium, or arsenic. In fact, all children's products, antacids, juices, and adult chewable products had less than 1 mcg of lead per gram of calcium, as did most of the other products. This level is well below the standard limit of 7.5 micrograms of lead per gram of calcium.

QUALITY PRODUCTS
Listed alphabetically by name on pages 86 to 89 are the products that passed ConsumerLab.com's independent testing of calcium dietary supplements (see Calcium approved-quality products).

CONSUMERTIPS™ FOR BUYING AND USING
ConsumerLab.com has prepared numerous important tips about dosing, selecting, and buying calcium supplements. This information — along with our list of approved-quality brands — provides a valuable guide for choosing appropriate products.

The following information about recommended intakes will help you determine which amounts are appropriate for your gender and life stage. Remember that 1,000 mcg (micrograms) equals 1 mg (milligram) and that 1,000 mg equals 1 gram. (See Understanding Recommended Dietary Allowances, Adequate Intakes, Tolerable Upper Intake Levels, page 46.)

Of the products evaluated, calcium content ranged from 125 to 600 mg/tablet and 345 to 500 mg/soft chew, tablespoon of liquid, or glass of juice, according to the labels. When comparing the costs of calcium products, consider the calcium amount per serving. Labels should indicate the amount of elemental calcium per dose because calcium actually makes up less than half of the weight of calcium compounds. For example, only 40% of the weight of calcium carbonate is calcium, as is only 9% of the weight of calcium gluconate.

Recommended daily intake: The recommended adequate intake

of calcium as determined by National Academy of Sciences varies by age. For adults ages 19 to 50, the recommended daily intake is 1,000 mg; for adults older than age 50, it's 1,200 mg. The National Institutes of Health recommends that postmenopausal women not taking estrogen get 1,500 mg. For younger individuals, the recommended amounts are 1,300 mg for those ages 9 through 18; 800 mg for children ages 4 to 8; and 500 mg for children ages 1 to 3. Although the recommended intake of calcium isn't higher during pregnancy or breast-feeding (because women's bodies are better able to absorb and maintain calcium during these times), intake should be met to support proper bone density in the fetus.

The AI for calcium is 500 mg for children ages 1 to 3, 800 mg for children ages 4 to 8, and 1,300 mg for individuals ages 9 to 18. For adults ages 19 to 50, the RDA is 1,000 mg. For adults ages 51 and older, it's 1,200 mg/day. The National Institutes of Health recommends 1,500 mg/day for postmenopausal women not taking hormone replacement therapy.

Upper limit: Too much calcium can contribute to kidney failure as well as excessive bone formation in children. The UL for calcium is 2,500 mg and applies to all individuals ages 1 and older.

Remember, the recommended amounts are for total daily calcium intake from food sources and supplementation. Note: An 8-ounce cup of milk or yogurt provides almost 300 mg of calcium; a cup of cottage cheese or ice cream, less than 200 mg. Other foods such as white beans, tofu, and broccoli provide smaller amounts.

When taking calcium supplements, divide the doses during the day so that no more than 500 mg is taken at time.

CAUTIONS AND CONCERNS

Calcium is safe when taken in the recommended amounts, but be aware that combined calcium intake from food and supplements shouldn't exceed 2,500 mg/day, experts say.

Calcium approved-quality products

Product name Manufacturer (Mf) or distributor (Dist)	Calcium (mg)/unit	Form of calcium
Adult tablets (nonchewable)		
Calcimate Plus 800 *Dist: GNC*	200 mg/tablet	calcium citrate malate
Calcium Magnesium Plus Phosphorus and Vitamin D *Dist: Shaklee Corp.*	162.5 mg/tablet	dicalcium phosphate
Calcium Xtra with Soy Isoflavones, Vitamin D and Minerals *Dist: Sundown*	600 mg/tablet	calcium carbonate
Caltrate® 600 Plus Calcium Dietary Supplement with Vitamin D and Minerals‡ *Marketed by Whitehall-Robins Healthcare*	600 mg/tablet	calcium carbonate
Citracal® Calcium Citrate Ultradense *Dist: Mission Pharmacal*	200 mg/tablet	calcium citrate
Fields of Nature Natural Calcium, Magnesium, and Zinc *Dist: Fields of Nature*	333.3 mg/tablet	calcium carbonate
Nature Made Calcium and Magnesium with Zinc‡ *Dist: Nature Made Nutritional Products*	333 mg/tablet	calcium carbonate
Nature's Bounty Calcium Citrate *Mf: Nature's Bounty*	200 mg/tablet	calcium citrate
Nutrilite® Calcium Magnesium Plus‡ *Mf: Nutrilite, a division of Amway Corp.*	217 mg/tablet	calcium carbonate
One A Day Women's Multivitamin/ Multimineral Supplement *Dist: Bayer*	450 mg/tablet	calcium carbonate

Product name Manufacturer (Mf) or distributor (Dist)	Calcium (mg)/unit	Form of calcium
Os Cal Calcium Supplement *Dist: SmithKline Beecham Consumer* *Healthcare, L.P.*	500 mg/tablet	oyster shell
Posture-D Calcium Supplement with Vitamin D *Dist: Inverness Medical, Inc.*	600 mg/tablet	tribasic calcium phosphate
Puritan's Pride Calcium Citrate *Mf: Puritan's Pride*	200 mg/tablet	calcium citrate
Schiff® Super Calcium 1200 With Vitamin D *Dist: Schiff®*	600 mg/softgel	calcium carbonate
Spring Valley Natural Oyster Shell Calcium 500 mg with Vitamin D *Mf: Perrigo*	500 mg/tablet	calcium carbonate
Vita-Smart Calcium Oyster Shell With Vitamin D *Mf: for Kmart*	500 mg/tablet	calcium carbonate
Walgreens Pharmaceutical Grade Calcium Magnesium *Dist: Walgreen Co.*	333 mg/caplet	calcium carbonate
Your Life Natural Oyster Shell Calcium with Vitamin D *Dist: Leiner Health Products Inc.*	500 mg/tablet	oyster shell

Soft Chewable

CalBurst Calcium Supplement‡ *Mf: Nature Made Nutritional Products*	500 mg/soft chew	calcium carbonate
Viactiv Calcium Supplement plus Vitamins D and K *Dist: Mead Johnson Nutritionals,* *A Bristol-Myers Squibb Company*	500 mg/soft chew	calcium carbonate

(continued)

Calcium

Product name Manufacturer (Mf) or distributor (Dist)	Calcium (mg)/unit	Form of calcium
Antacids		
Extra Strength Mylanta Calci Tabs Antacid/Calcium Supplement *Dist: Johnson & Johnson Merck*	300 mg/chewable tablet	calcium carbonate
Extra Strength Rolaids Antacid *Dist: Warner-Lambert Co.*	271 mg/chewable tablet	calcium carbonate
Quick Dissolve Maalox Maximum Strength Antacid/Calcium Supplement *Dist: Novartis Consumer Health, Inc.*	370 mg/chewable tablet	calcium carbonate
Tums 500 Calcium Supplement *Dist: SmithKline Beecham Consumer Healthcare, L.P.*	500 mg/chewable tablet	calcium carbonate
Foods with added calcium		
Minute Maid Premium Original Plus Calcium Orange Juice *Dist: The Minute Maid Company, a Division of the Coca-Cola Company*	350 mg/240 mL liquid	tricalcium phosphate, calcium lactate
Tropicana Pure Premium Calcium and Vitamin C Enriched Orange Juice *Dist: Tropicana Products, Inc.*	350 mg/240 mL liquid	FruitCal® (calcium hydroxide)
Children's supplements		
Centrum Kids with Extra Calcium and Shamu and His Crew‡ *Marketed by Whitehall-Robins Healthcare*	200 mg/chewable tablet	calcium carbonate calcium phosphate
Flintstones Plus Calcium Children's Multivitamin Plus Calcium Supplement *Dist: Bayer Corp.*	200 mg/chewable tablet	calcium carbonate

Product name Manufacturer (Mf) or distributor (Dist)	Calcium (mg)/unit	Form of calcium
GNC Kids Multibite™ plus minerals and *Dist: GNC*	200 mg/chewable tablet and calcium	calcium carbonate dicalcium phosphate
Naturally Kids' Calcees *Dist: Naturally Vitamins* calcium	300 mg/chewable tablet	calcium carbonate, calcium citrate, gluconate, calcium amino acid chelate
Nature's Plus Animal Parade Children's Chewable Calcium Supplement *Mf: Natural Organics Laboratories, Inc.*	125 mg/chewable tablet	Aminoate complex

‡ See "More Brand Information," page 191.

Iron

WHAT IT IS

Iron, an essential mineral that the body requires in small amounts, is widely distributed in foods including meat, poultry, fish, dried fruits, grains, and green leafy vegetables. Iron from plant sources is absorbed half as well as that from animal sources. The average diet provides 10 to 20 mg of iron per day.

WHAT IT DOES

Iron is needed to manufacture hemoglobin, which enables red blood cells to transfer oxygen to the body's tissues. Iron deficiency is the leading cause of anemia, which can lead to lethargy and fatigue, and if severe enough, death. Deficiency is most common in menstruating women but is also commonly seen in children and pregnant women. Low iron levels may also result from excessive bleeding, burns, and hemodialysis as well as stomach and intestinal problems. During pregnancy, iron deficiency can result in preterm delivery and low-birth-weight babies. Among children, iron deficiency is most common from ages 6 to 24 months, where it can cause irreversible developmental and behavioral problems. At the other end of the spectrum, too much iron can be toxic and is a leading cause of poisoning in children. Some preliminary research, however, suggests that high-dose iron supplements may be helpful in reducing the dry cough caused by angiotensin-converting enzyme inhibitors.

QUALITY CONCERNS

How much iron should a supplement contain? That's difficult to say. People's needs and diets vary; hence, the amount of supplementation necessary varies. At this time, there's no established standard, and the amount varies widely among brands. Moreover, iron is available in many forms. All can supply adequate iron, although absorption and adverse effects may vary.

Because no government agency is responsible for routinely testing iron supplements for their contents or quality, Consumerlab.com independently evaluated several leading iron products to determine whether they contained the iron types and amounts stated on their labels. The products were also tested for disintegration and contamination with lead—a harmful contaminant found in some mineral supplements. In fact, in 1997, the U.S. Food and Drug Administration (FDA) reported that several iron-containing supplements had been recalled because of excessive levels of lead.

PRODUCT TESTING

ConsumerLab.com purchased 19 iron supplements and tested them for their amount of iron, disintegration, and contamination with lead. (See "ConsumerLab.com's testing methods and standards," page 169.)

TEST FINDINGS

ConsumerLab.com purchased 19 iron supplements, several of which included other nutrients, such as vitamin C, folic acid and other B vitamins, various herbs, and calcium.

Of these 19 products, 17 passed all criteria. Of the 2 that didn't pass, 1 product—a store-brand supplement from a major pharmacy chain—had only 73% of its claimed 27 mg of iron per capsule. The other product didn't pass because it contained lead at a level in excess of 0.5 mcg/day. This product, from a national manufacturer, contained additional vitamins and herbs and was specifically marketed for use by women. Most lead poisoning results from multiple exposures over time, and though the level found in this supplement doesn't represent an immediate threat in itself, it unnecessarily contributes to daily lead exposure. The other iron products tested contained far lower or undetectable levels of lead in a daily dose.

Iron approved-quality products

Product name (iron form, elemental iron/unit)	Manufacturer (Mf) or distributor (Dist)
Country Life Target-Mins (ferrous aspartate, 25 mg/tablet)	Dist: Country Life
Feosol Ferrous Sulfate (ferrous sulfate, 65 mg/tablet)	Dist: SmithKline Beecham Consumer Healthcare, L.P.
Fergon Ferrous Gluconate (ferrous gluconate, 27 mg/tablet)	Dist: Bayer Corporation
Ferro-Sequels (ferrous fumarate, 50 mg/tablet)	Dist: Inverness Medical, Inc.
Good Neighbor Pharmacy Ferrous Sulfate (ferrous sulfate, 65 mg/tablet)	Dist: Bergen Brunswig Drug Company
Nature Made® Iron Supplement (ferrous sulfate, 65 mg/tablet)*	Dist: Nature Made Nutritional Products
Nature's Bounty Ferrous Gluconate (ferrous gluconate, 28 mg/tablet)	Mf: Nature's Bounty Inc.
Nature's Bounty Ferrous Sulfate (ferrous sulfate, 28 mg/tablet)	Mf: Nature's Bounty Inc.
Nutrilite Iron-Folic Plus (ferrous fumarate, 15 mg/tablet)‡	Dist: Access Business Group International LLC
Puritan's Pride Iron All Organic Iron Plus Liver, B Complex, Vitamin C, Iron and Multivitamin Supplement (ferrous gluconate, 19.2 mg/tablet)	Mfd. for Puritan's Pride Inc.
Safeway Select Iron (ferrous sulfate, 27 mg/tablet)	Dist: Safeway Inc.
Slow Fe Slow Release Iron (ferrous sulfate, 50 mg/tablet)	Dist: Novartis Consumer Health, Inc.
Solaray Iron (iron acid chelate, 50 mg/capsule)	Mf: Nutraceutical Corp. for Solaray Inc.
Sundown Perfect Iron (carbonyl iron, 25 mg/tablet)	Mf: Sundown Vitamins
Twinlab Iron Caps (ferrous fumarate, 18 mg/capsule)	Mf: Twin Laboratories Inc.
Vitamin World Easy Iron (Iron Glycinate) (iron bis-glycinate, 28 mg/capsule)	Mf: Vitamin World
Vitasmart Iron (Ferrous Sulfate) (ferrous sulfate, 27 mg/tablet)	Dist: Kmart Corp.

Product name (iron form, elemental iron/unit)	Manufacturer (Mf) or distributor (Dist)
Whole Foods Chelated Iron (ferrous bis-glycinate, 18 mg/capsule)	Mf: Whole Foods Market

* Tested through ConsumerLab.com's Ad Hoc Testing Program (Product was tested at the manufacturer's request after the initial review was completed and released.)

‡ See "More Brand Information," page 191.

QUALITY PRODUCTS

Listed alphabetically by name on the previous page are the products that passed ConsumerLab.com's independent testing of iron dietary supplements (see Iron approved-quality products). Note: Many of the products may have been designed for treating iron deficiency and, therefore, exceed the Recommended Dietary Allowance (RDA) as well as the tolerable upper intake level (UL) for iron. Under a physician's supervision it's acceptable to exceed these limits, because the potential consequences of untreated iron deficiency may be more severe than the potential adverse effects of high iron intake.

CONSUMERTIPS™ FOR BUYING AND USING

ConsumerLab.com has prepared numerous important tips about dosing, selecting, and buying iron supplements. This information — along with our list of approved-quality brands — provides a valuable guide for choosing appropriate products.

The following information will help you determine which amounts are appropriate for your gender and life stage. Remember that 1,000 mcg (micrograms) equals 1 mg (milligram) and that 1,000 mg equals 1 gram.

The FDA requires that dietary supplements state on their labels the % Daily Value for certain vitamins and minerals. However, the percentages given may not reflect the latest RDAs or Adequate Intakes (AIs). Moreover, the labels are unlikely to provide information indicating whether the ingredients exceed ULs — as many do — because the FDA doesn't require that information. (See Understanding

Recommended Dietary Allowances, Adequate Intakes, Tolerable Upper Intake Levels, page 46.)

Several different forms of iron are used in supplements. Fortunately, the consumer doesn't need to convert the percentages of weight to elemental iron; the manufacturer does this, and the appropriate amount appears on the label. Generally, the least expensive forms are ferrous (iron) sulfate, ferrous fumarate, and ferrous gluconate.

Men ages 18 and older and postmenopausal women (if not taking hormone replacement therapy) rarely experience iron-deficiency anemia (low iron); therefore, there's little reason for these groups to take an iron supplement. For individuals diagnosed with iron-deficiency anemia, the recommended dose depends on the severity of the anemia and should be determined by a physician. In general, however, the daily dose for mild to moderate anemia is about 60 mg of elemental iron from ferrous sulfate (or ferrous fumarate or ferrous gluconate) for about 2 months, to improve hemoglobin level. Therapy may continue for another 2 months to build up iron stores.

Recommended daily intake: The RDA for iron is 7 mg for children ages 1 to 3 and 10 mg for children ages 4 to 8. It then decreases to 8 mg for children ages 9 to 13. For males ages 14 to 18, the RDA is 11 mg, and for males ages 19 and older, it decreases to 8 mg. For females, ages 14 to 18, it's 15 mg, and for ages 19 to 50, it's 18 mg, decreasing to 8 mg for women ages 51 and older. Because of fetal needs, the RDA for pregnant women is to 27 mg. For breast-feeding women younger than age 18, the RDA is 10 mg; for breast-feeding women ages 19 and older, it's 9 mg. Also, postmenopausal women taking hormone replacement therapy should consume more iron because the therapy can cause periodic uterine bleeding. Oral contraceptives may reduce menstrual blood loss, so women taking them may need less daily iron.

Upper limit: High daily amounts of iron can cause gastrointestinal distress, especially when iron supplements are consumed on an empty stomach. The UL is 40 mg for children younger than age 13, and 45 mg for everyone else. However, these limits may be too high for people with hereditary hemochromatosis, who are at risk for accumulating harmful levels of iron.

If you have difficulty tolerating iron tablets, consider chelated iron, time-release iron supplements, ferrous bisglycinate, or ferrous glycinate, all of which are fairly expensive but may be the least likely to cause a stomach upset. Another form, carbonyl iron, may present a reduced risk of harm in an accidental overdose. Carbonyl iron is, consequently, the ingredient many children's supplements contain and may be preferred by parents of small children. Injectable iron is also available under the supervision of a health professional.

Still another way to deal with gastric upset is to take an iron supplement with food. Though combining the supplement with food may decrease iron absorption, taking it with a vitamin C–rich food may offset that effect; vitamin C boosts iron absorption. In fact, some iron supplements contain vitamin C as an added ingredient to aid absorption. Also, remember that many antacids can decrease iron absorption, as can soy protein, coffee, tea, eggs, whole-grain cereals and breads, spinach, and calcium. When consuming one of these foods, wait 1 to 2 hours to take your iron supplement.

CAUTIONS AND CONCERNS

Iron is safe when taken in appropriate amounts, but be aware that high daily amounts of supplemental iron can cause gastrointestinal distress, especially if it's taken on an empty stomach.

When taken continually, iron can result in toxicity, causing cirrhosis, coronary heart disease, congestive heart failure, and other problems. Toxicity is a major concern for individuals with hemochromatosis, a genetic condition affecting 1 out of every 200 to 500 people. With hemochromatosis, excessive amounts of iron build up in the body's tissues and organs.

Iron supplements may reduce the absorption of certain drugs such as levodopa, levothyroxine, penicillamine, quinolone antibiotics, and tetracycline antibiotics. Some of these drugs may, conversely, interfere with iron absorption.

Remember, iron supplements are a leading cause of poisoning in children younger than age 6 (just a few adult tablets can cause serious poisoning), so keep iron products away from children's reach. To help reduce the number of such poisonings, supplements containing 30 mg or more of iron (other than carbonyl iron) can be sold only in child-resistant bottles or in single-dose packaging.

PART THREE

Product reviews for herbals and other supplements

Coenzyme Q10

WHAT IT IS

Coenzyme Q10 (CoQ10), also known as ubiquinone, is a naturally occurring body compound used for energy production within cells. It's manufactured in the heart, liver, kidney, and pancreas. The body normally produces sufficient CoQ10, although some medications may interfere with this process and CoQ10 levels in the body may decline with age and heart disease. Only small amounts of CoQ10 are available from food, mainly beef and chicken. Consequently, dietary supplements are the most common way to increase the body's CoQ10 levels.

WHAT IT DOES

Coenzyme Q10 may help treat congestive heart failure, a disease in which the heart doesn't adequately maintain circulation. CoQ10 plays a role in cell energy production, and this may be the mechanism by which it assists the heart. Although the evidence is weak, CoQ10's role as an antioxidant may also be useful for treating other diseases affecting the heart muscle as well as for healing periodontal infections, muscular dystrophy, Huntington's disease, AIDS, hypertension, and some cancers. The role of CoQ10 in enhancing athletic performance hasn't been well demonstrated.

QUALITY CONCERNS

Because no government agency is responsible for routinely testing CoQ10 supplements or other dietary supplements for their contents or quality, ConsumerLab.com independently evaluated several leading CoQ10 products to determine whether they contained the amounts of CoQ10 stated on their labels.

PRODUCT TESTING

ConsumerLab.com purchased 29 different CoQ10 products, several of which also contained other ingredients, such as bioflavonoids and vitamin E. The group contained these products: 17 softgels, 11 tablets or capsules, and 1 sublingual tablet. These products were tested for their claimed amount of CoQ10. (See "ConsumerLab.com's testing methods and standards," page 169.)

TEST FINDINGS

Of the 29 products tested, 1 product, a capsule that had no more than 17% of its stated CoQ10, failed testing.

QUALITY PRODUCTS

Listed alphabetically by name on pages 101 to 102 are the products that passed ConsumerLab.com's independent testing of CoQ10 dietary supplements (see CoQ10 approved-quality products).

CONSUMERTIPS™ FOR BUYING AND USING

ConsumerLab.com has prepared numerous important tips about dosing, selecting, and buying CoQ10 supplements. This information — along with our list of approved-quality brands — provides a valuable guide for choosing appropriate products.

CoQ10 recommended daily dosages vary widely, resulting in products on the market that claim to contain anywhere from 10 to 120 mg/pill of the substance. When comparing product costs, consider the dosage and number of pills per bottle.

Using CoQ10 to treat congestive heart failure should be considered an adjunct to, not a replacement for, other medications; a daily dose of 100 to 200 mg of CoQ10 is generally used, with the dose depending on the individual's weight. Be aware that improvement in symptoms may take more than 1 month. Don't suddenly stop taking CoQ10, because symptoms may worsen. Tapering off the supplement is recommended.

CoQ10 approved-quality products

Product name (amount of CoQ10/pill, type)	Manufacturer (Mf) or Distributor (Dist)
Carlson® CoQ10 (50 mg/softgel)	Dist: Carlson, Division of J.R. Carlson Laboratories, Inc.
CVS® Coenzyme Q10 Dietary Supplement (50 mg/capsule)	Dist: CVS Pharmacy, Inc.
Fields of Nature® LiquafilTM Softgels CoEnzyme Q-10, (30 mg/EZ to Swallow)	Dist: Fields of Nature, Div. of IVC Industries, Inc.
Gary Null's New & Improved Super Coenzyme Q10 Dietary Supplement (100 mg/tablet)	Dist: Gary Null & Associates
GNC Preventive Nutrition® Coenzyme Q-10 Dietary Supplement (30 mg/softgel)	Dist: General Nutrition Corporation
Natrol® CoEnzyme Q-10 30 mg Dietary Supplement (30 mg/capsule)	Mf: Natrol
Nature Made® CoQ10 100 mg Dietary Supplement (100 mg/softgel)* ‡	Dist: Nature Made
Nature's Bounty® Q-SorbTM Coenzyme Q10 30 mg Dietary Supplement (30 mg/softgel)	Mf: Nature's Bounty, Inc.
Nature's Bounty® Q-SorbTM Coenzyme Q10 50 mg Dietary Supplement (50 mg/softgel)	Mf: Nature's Bounty, Inc.
Nature's Plus®, The Energy Supplements® Ultra CoQ10 Maximum Strength (100 mg/softgel)	Dist: Nature's Plus, Div. of Natural Organics, Inc.
Nature's Way® CoQ10 60 mg Improved Absorption Dietary Supplement (60 mg/softgel)	Dist: Nature's Way Products, Inc.
Now® CoQ10 30 mg, Highest Quality (capsule)	Dist: Now Foods
Nutrilite Coenzyme Q10 dietary supplement (30 mg/capsule) ‡	Mf: Nutrilite, a division of Access Business Group International LLC
Puritan's Pride® Inspired By NatureTM CoenzymeQ-10 10 mg Dietary Supplement (softgel)	Mf: Puritan's Pride, Inc.
Schiff® CoQ-10 (Coenzyme Q-10) Dietary Supplement (30 mg/capsule)	Dist: Schiff Products, Inc.

(continued)

Product name (amount of CoQ10/pill, type)	Manufacturer (Mf) or Distributor (Dist)
Solaray® Dietary Supplement Fortified CoQ-10 (30 mg/capsule)	Mf: Nutraceutical Corp. for Solaray, Inc.
Solgar CoQ-10 (Coenzyme Q-10) 30 mg Dietary Supplement (30 mg/capsule)	Mf: Solgar Vitamin and Herb
Source Naturals® Coenzyme Q10 Antioxidant Support Dietary Supplement (30 mg/sublingual tablet)	Dist: Source Naturals, Inc.
Sundown® Natural Coenzyme Q-10 (30 mg/softgel)	Dist: Distribution by Sundown Vitamins
TruNature® Coenzyme Q10 Specialty Supplement (50 mg/softgel)	Dist: Leiner Health Products, Inc.
TwinLab® Mega CoQ10TM (Coenzyme Q10) Dietary Supplement (30 mg/capsule)	Mf: Twin Laboratories Inc.
Q-Gel Coenzyme Q-10 (15 mg/softgel)	Mf: Gel-Tec, Div. of Tishcon Corp.
Q-Gel® Forte Coenzyme Q-10 (30 mg/softgel)	Mf: Gel-Tec, Div. of Tishcon Corp.
Q-Gel® Ultra Coenzyme Q-10 (60 mg, softgel)	Mf: Gel-Tec, Div. of Tishcon Corp.
Q-Gel® Plus Coenzyme Q-10 30 mg Plus Alpha Lipoic Acid and Vitamin E (30 mg/softgel)	Mf: Gel-Tec, Div. of Tishcon Corp.
The Vitamin Shoppe® Coenzyme Q-10, 75 mg (75 mg, capsule)	Dist: The Vitamin Shoppe
Vitamin World® Naturally InspiredTM Coenzyme Q-10 75 mg Dietary Supplement (75 mg/softgel).	Mf: Vitamin World, Inc.
Vitamin World® Naturally InspiredTM Coenzyme Q-10 120 mg Dietary Supplement (120 mg/softgel)	Mf: Vitamin World, Inc.
Your Life® Coenzyme Q10 30 mg Supplement (30 mg/softgel)	Dist: Leiner Health Products, Inc.

* Tested through ConsumerLab.com's Ad Hoc Testing Program (Product was tested at the manufacturer's request after the initial review was completed and released.)
‡ See "More Brand Information," page 191.

For conditions other than congestive heart failure, daily doses as low as 30 mg and as high as 300 mg have also been used.

Divided dosing (taking two small doses instead of one large dose a day) is recommended when the total daily dose exceeds 100 mg.

CoQ10, especially the dry dosage form (tablet or capsule), is best absorbed when fats or oils are present in the gastrointestinal tract, so take the supplement with meals. A softgel isn't considered a dry form.

CAUTIONS AND CONCERNS

CoQ10 is generally safe when taken in appropriate amounts, but be aware of that CoQ10's safety has not been evaluated for children and pregnant or breast-feeding women.

Individuals with diabetes and those taking blood thinners are strongly advised to consult a physician before taking this supplement, because of potential drug interactions.

Certain medications, including some cholesterol-lowering statin drugs, beta-blockers, antidepressants, and antipsychotics may decrease the body's natural production of CoQ10; therefore, the CoQ10 dosage for individuals taking any of these drugs should possibly be higher than generally recommended.

Creatine

WHAT IT IS

Creatine (creatine monohydrate) is made up of three amino acids: glycine, arginine, and methionine. Creatine phosphate, which is produced by the body and found in muscle, supplies energy for short-term, maximal exercise. Food sources of creatine include meat, poultry, and fish.

WHAT IT DOES

Creatine is used in the United States as a sports supplement. Used appropriately, it can, according to some studies, improve performance during high-intensity exercise of short duration, such as weight lifting and sprinting.

QUALITY CONCERNS

When creatine is metabolized in the body, it creates a waste product called "creatinine," which is normally removed from the body by the kidneys. (Blood levels of creatinine are commonly used to evaluate kidney functioning). Creatinine also appears in impure creatine supplements as a result of improper manufacturing or breakdown of the creatine, as does another manufacturing by-product, dicyandiamide. Although creatinine and dicyandiamide in small amounts don't appear to pose a safety risk, they aren't useful and must be eliminated through the kidneys. Hence, manufacturers like to claim their products are "100% pure," "99% pure," or "dicyandiamide free" because quality creatine shouldn't contain these impurities. Purity has become an issue because creatine dosages are relatively large—sometimes exceeding 20 grams/day (about 4 tsp of creatine powder).

Because no government agency is responsible for routinely testing creatine supplements for their contents or quality, ConsumerLab.com has independently evaluated several leading creatine products to determine whether they possessed the quality and amount of creatine stated on their labels. It also tested to determine whether the products were contaminated with creatinine or dicyandiamide.

PRODUCT TESTING
ConsumerLab.com purchased 13 brands of creatine monohydrate supplements. The products were tested for creatine monohydrate and contamination with creatinine and dicyandiamide. (See "ConsumerLab.com's testing methods and standards," page 169.)

TEST FINDINGS
Of the 13 creatine monohydrate brands tested, 11 passed the evaluation. Of the products that failed, 1 contained less than the labeled amount of creatine and the other didn't meet its dicyandiamide-free claim.

QUALITY PRODUCTS
Listed alphabetically by name on page 106 are the products that passed ConsumerLab.com's independent testing of creatine dietary supplements (see Creatine approved-quality products).

CONSUMERTIPS™ FOR BUYING AND USING
ConsumerLab.com has prepared numerous important tips about dosing, selecting, and buying creatine supplements. This information — along with our list of approved-quality brands — provides a valuable guide for choosing appropriate products.

Ideally, product labels should indicate the product contains pure "creatine monohydrate" and state the amount in the container or dosage form (for example, powder [typically mixed with water or juice], drink mix, capsules, or tablets). Consider the dosage when comparing product costs. Among the products evaluated, the labeled amount of creatine monohydrate ranged from 100 to 500 grams of powder per scoop; tablets and capsules contained from 700 to 1,000 mg.

Creatine monohydrate approved-quality products

Product name (form and concentration of creatine pills)	Manufacturer (Mf) and/or distributor (Dist)
99% Pure Creatine - Creatine Monohydrate (powder)	Mf: Natrol, Inc.
Athletic Series Creatine (1,000 mg/tablet)	Dist: Source Naturals, Inc.
Body Fortress® Hardcore Formula Creatine Powder HPLC*	Mf: U.S. Nutrition
Body Fortress® High Performance Creatine, Grape Flavor (powder)*	Dist: U.S. Nutrition
Creapure™ Creatine Monohydrate Powder	Mf: Prolab Nutrition
Creatine 6000-ES Creatine Monohydrate (powder)	Dist: Muscletech Research and Development
Creatine Monohydrate (725 mg/capsule)	Dist: Weider Nutrition International
Creatine Monohydrate (powder)	Mf: SportPharma USA, Inc.
Engineered Nutrition Micronized Creatine 99% Pure (powder)	Dist: Met-Rx
High-Energy Creatine Loading Formula Universal Micronized Creatine, Creapure™ 100% Pure Creatine Monohydrate (powder)	Mf: Universal Nutrition
Perfect Creatine Monohydrate (powder)	Dist: Nature's Best
Performance Enhancer Creatine Fuel (700 mg/capsule)	Mf: Twin Laboratories, Inc.
Phosphagen™—Pure Creatine Monohydrate (powder)	Dist: EAS®
Precision Engineered™ Hardcore Formula Creatine Caps (700 mg/capsule)*	Mf: U.S. Nutrition
Precision Engineered™ Hardcore Formula Creatine Powder*	Mf: U.S. Nutrition
Precision Engineered™ High Performance Creatine HPDS3 High Performance DeliverySystem Third Generation, Fruit Punch Flavor (powder)*	Dist: U.S. Nutrition

* Tested through ConsumerLab.com's Ad Hoc Testing Program (Product was tested at the manufacturer's request after the initial review was completed and released.)

Copyright ConsumerLab.com, LLC, 2000, 2001, 2002, 2003. All rights reserved. Not to be reproduced, excerpted, or cited without written permission from ConsumerLab.com LLC.

Dosing regimens are designed to increase the levels of creatine, in its storage form, in muscle tissue. The standard dose is 2 to 5 grams of creatine per day. On this dosing regimen, the maximum creatine storage should occur within 2 to 4 weeks. For more rapid increases, 20 to 25 grams/day (in four divided doses of 5 to 6 grams throughout each day) is taken for the first 5 days.

CAUTIONS AND CONCERNS

Creatine is generally considered safe when taken in appropriate amounts, but be aware that it may cause muscle cramping, diarrhea, and dehydration in some people, according to reports. Also, high doses (20 grams/day) over long periods may cause kidney disease, and little is known about other potential long-term adverse effects.

Creatine supplements may be dangerous for people with existing kidney disease.

Creatine's safety during pregnancy and breast-feeding hasn't been evaluated; therefore, use of the supplement isn't recommended at those times.

Echinacea

WHAT IT IS

Echinacea, a popular herb, is used primarily to reduce the symptoms and duration of colds and flulike illnesses.

There are three species of Echinacea: E. purpurea, E. angustifolia, and E. pallida. Supplements may be made from the aboveground (or aerial) or root portions of echinacea, depending on the species, although it's unclear which of the herb's many chemical components is responsible for its effects. However, the Echinacea species does appear to possess marker compounds for a chemical class called "phenols." For example, the aerial and root portions of E. purpurea contain cichoric and caftaric acid phenols; E. angustifolia and E. pallida roots, the echinacoside phenol. These compounds can, then, become markers to evaluate the quality of an echinacea product.

WHAT IT DOES

Echinacea appears to work through short-term stimulation of the immune system. It hasn't, however, been proven effective in preventing disease and isn't recommended for long-term use, which may actually depress the immune system.

QUALITY CONCERNS

Microbes can contaminate herbal products during growing, harvesting, or production. Unfortunately, the presence of microbes can also indicate plant material decomposition. As a result, the World Health Organization (WHO) has established standards for microbial contamination of medicinal plant materials intended for internal use, and the U.S. Food and Drug Administration (FDA) has established zero tolerance levels for certain disease-causing bacteria.

Because no government agency is responsible for routinely testing echinacea products, ConsumerLab.com has independently evaluated several leading echinacea products for their quality and quantity of Echinacea. It has also tested for levels of microbial contamination.

PRODUCT TESTING

ConsumerLab.com purchased 25 echinacea products and tested them for 100% of the claimed amounts and types of echinacea, as well as the claimed levels of phenols (specifically caftaric acid, chlorogenic acid, echinacoside, and cichoric acid). If the phenol levels weren't clearly labeled, products were held to specific minimum standards consistent with clinical research on echinacea. Products were also required to meet purity requirements for microbial contamination. (See "ConsumerLab.com's testing methods and standards," page 169.)

TEST FINDINGS

Of the 25 echinacea products purchased, 6 were eliminated from testing because of inadequate ingredient labeling. Specifically, 3 products didn't identify the species of Echinacea, 1 product didn't state the part of the plant used, and 2 liquids, or tinctures, didn't state the concentration of echinacea. Since March 1999, the FDA has required that herbal product labels provide such information.

Among the remaining 19 products, 12 claimed to contain only E. purpurea, 2 claimed to contain only E. angustifolia, and 5 were mixtures of two or more species of Echinacea. Some products also contained other ingredients, such as goldenseal. Only 3 products tested specifically indicated the levels of phenols they contained.

Of the 19 products tested, 5 didn't pass the evaluations: 2 of the 12 E. purpurea–only products tested failed. One, an extract made from aerial portions of the plant, had only 54% of the minimum expected phenol levels. The other, a root powder, had nearly three times the acceptable level of microbes set by WHO. The microbes were aerobic bacteria, indicative of decomposition (not coliform bacteria, associated with fecal contamination). The other 10 E. purpurea products that passed were made from aerial portions of the herb (flower, leaves, and stems).

Both E. angustifolia–only products failed. One, made from root powder, had no detectable levels of echinacoside, a known marker for this species. The other, a root extract, had less than one-third of the 4% phenol content claimed.

One combination product failed because it lacked detectable levels of echinacoside, although it claimed to contain E. angustifolia root extract.

In summary, of the 25 products originally purchased, only 14 products (56%) passed ConsumerLab.com's review. It's possible that the products that didn't contain the expected levels of markers were made from other types of echinacea or, perhaps, contained other ingredients altogether.

QUALITY PRODUCTS
Listed alphabetically by name on pages 112 to 113 are the products that passed ConsumerLab.com's independent testing of Echinacea dietary supplements (see Echinacea approved-quality products).

CONSUMERTIPS™ FOR BUYING AND USING
ConsumerLab.com has prepared numerous important tips about dosing, selecting, and buying echinacea supplements. This information — along with our list of approved-quality brands — provides a valuable guide for choosing appropriate products.

Label information as required by the FDA should appear on all echinacea product labels (see "Passing score," page 179). In addition, the concentration of total phenols should be indicated; this information is a marker for the quality of the echinacea in the product. The total phenolic content should be at least 1% for whole herb or root products and should be proportionally higher for extracts and tinctures, depending on the concentration.

Most clinical studies showing benefit from echinacea use have been conducted with products made from the aerial portions of E. purpurea or the root portion of E. pallida. However, the United States Pharmacopoeia also recognizes the use of roots from E. purpurea and E. angustifolia. All the products (10 out of 10) made from E. purpurea — specifically prepared from aerial plant portions (flower, leaves, and stems) and made directly from the whole herb (as opposed to an extract) — passed ConsumerLab.com's review.

Echinacea products come in many forms and concentrations; therefore, the dosage varies depending on the product. The standard dose of echinacea extract (generally a 4x concentration) is 900 mg/day in three doses of 300 mg each. For products made from the whole herb or root, the dosage is 1 to 2 grams three times per day. As an alcohol tincture (5x concentration), 3 to 4 ml are generally taken three times per day.

Treatment should start at the first sign of a cold and continue for 1 to 2 weeks. However, treatment for more than 8 weeks should be avoided. Among the products evaluated, the manufacturers' recommended dosages of extract varied from 50 to 1,000 mg/day; dosage recommendations for whole herb-root products ranged from 1,000 to 8,000 mg/day. Consequently, it's best to compare the cost of equivalent daily doses rather than the number of daily servings per container.

Many echinacea products also contain goldenseal. Though goldenseal may be useful as an antibiotic when applied directly to an infection, it isn't useful for treating colds. Goldenseal shouldn't be used during pregnancy.

CAUTIONS AND CONCERNS

Uncontaminated echinacea is considered relatively safe when taken in appropriate amounts, but be aware that it does have some adverse effects, including minor gastrointestinal symptoms and increased urination.

Some people—especially those who are allergic to sunflowers and other flowers in the daisy family—may be allergic to echinacea. Also, because echinacea may affect the immune system, people with immune deficiencies or autoimmune diseases should avoid using this herb in any form.

The safety of echinacea hasn't been well established for children or for women who may become pregnant or who are pregnant or breast-feeding; therefore, individuals in these groups should avoid taking this herb.

Echinacea approved-quality products

Product name (amount and type of Echinacea/pill)	Manufacturer (Mf) or distributor (Dist)
CVS® Herbal Supplement Echinacea 380 mg Standardized (380 mg *Echinacea purpurea* herb powder)	Dist: CVS Pharmacy, Inc.
Frontier™ Certified Organic *Echinacea purpurea* Root Herbal Supplement (430 mg E. purpurea root powder)	Dist: Frontier
Health Pride, Immune System, Standardized Echinacea 380 mg Herbal Supplement (380 mg *E. purpurea* herb powder)	Dist: Compass Foods
Herbal Authority™ Echinacea 400 mg Herbal Supplement (400 mg *E. purpurea* root powder)	Mf: Herbal Authority, Div. of Puritan's Pride
NaturaLife® Total Release™ Herbs with digestive enzymes for absorption, Echinacea Standardized Extract & Whole Herb (190 mg *E. purpurea* [stem, leaf, flower] powder and 170 mg *E. angustifolia* root extract)]	Dist: NaturaLife Corp.
Naturally Preferred™ Certified Organic Herbal Supplement Echinacea Purpurea (380 mg *E. purpurea* herb powder)	Dist: Inter-American Products, Inc.
Nature's Bounty® Natural Echinacea 400 mg (400 mg *E. purpurea* root powder)	Mf: Nature's Bounty, Inc.
Nature's Way® Herbal Single Echinacea Herb (400 mg *E. purpurea* [stem, leaf, flower] powder)	Dist: Nature's Way Products Inc.
Nutrilite® Triple Guard Echinacea (168.7 mg *E. purpurea* root and aerial powder and *E. angustifolia* root powder) ‡	Mf: Nutrilite, a Division of Access Business Group International LLC
Nutrition Now® Chewable Echinacea Cold King™ (50 mg extract of *E. angustifolia* [root], *E. purpurea* [root], *E. pallida* [root and whole plant])	Dist: Nutrition Now Inc.
Optimum Nutrition Echinacea Purpurea (425 mg Aerial Powder)	Mf: Optimum Nutrition
Target™ Brand Echinacea Herbal Supplement (380 mg *E. purpurea* herb powder)	Dist: Target Corporation

(continued)

Echinacea

Product name (amount and type of Echinacea/pill)	Manufacturer (Mf) or distributor (Dist)
Tom's of Maine® Natural Echinacea Tonic With Green Tea Liquid Herbal Supplement, Ginger-Orange (1,015 mg/15 mL of E. purpurea [fresh root and dried aerial] powder, E. angustifolia [dried root] extract)	Dist: Tom's of Maine
TwinLab® TruHerbs® Echinacea Purpurea (400 mg E. purpurea herb powder)	Mf: Twin Laboratories Inc.

‡ See "More Brand Information," page 191.

Fish oils:
Omega-3 fatty acids
(EPA & DHA)

WHAT IT IS

Also known as omega-3 fatty acids, EPA (eicosapentaenoic acid) and DHA (docosahexaenoic acid) are the two principal fatty acids found in fish. Other marine sources, such as algae (algal oil), also contain DHA. EPA and DHA are polyunsaturated fats or "good" fats that don't increase the risk of heart disease. The body has a limited ability to manufacture EPA and DHA by converting the essential fatty acid alpha-linolenic acid (ALA), which is found in flaxseed oil, canola oil, and walnuts. But this ability is lessened if the diet is too high in omega-6 fatty acids, which come from vegetable oils, such as corn, sunflower, soybean, or safflower oil.

WHAT IT DOES

Omega-3 fatty acids (EPA and DHA) may help prevent heart disease and atherosclerosis by lowering triglyceride levels, raising high-density-lipoprotein ("good") cholesterol levels, and possibly "thinning" the blood. They may also reduce the risk of cardiac arrhythmias and one type of stroke. The U.S. Food and Drug Administration (FDA) now allows products containing omega-3 fatty acids to state: "The scientific evidence about whether omega-3 fatty acids may reduce the risk of coronary heart disease is suggestive, but not conclusive."

In addition, EPA and DHA can reduce the pain of rheumatoid arthritis by decreasing inflammation. The effect appears to help most in the early stages of arthritis, but it's unclear whether EPA and DHA affect the progression of the disease itself. Omega 3s may also reduce the pain associated with menstrual cramps.

Other conditions fish oils may help treat include bipolar (manic-depressive) disorder, Raynaud's phenomenon (abnormal sensitivity of hands and feet to cold), lupus, immunoglobulin A nephropathy, kidney stones, chronic fatigue syndrome, and cystic fibrosis. Fish oils were once considered potential therapy for ulcerative colitis and Crohn's disease, although more recent research hasn't shown benefits. In addition, omega 3s may reduce the risk of premature delivery in pregnant women and the risk of prostate cancer in men.

EPA specifically may be helpful for treating schizophrenia; DHA, for reducing high blood pressure. DHA is also important for normal development and functioning of the brain and retina in the fetus and in infants. The latter may explain the why infants of women who consume fish during pregnancy and while breast-feeding tend to have better vision. Consequently, DHA is often added to formula for premature infants and is also added to some regular infant formulas and foods. DHA may be helpful for treating disorders such as attention deficit, dyslexia, and cognitive impairment and dementia.

Moreover, experts now believe that the American diet contains too little of the omega-3 fatty acids and too much of the omega-6 fatty acids—and too much of the latter may increase the risk of heart disease and cancer. The ratio of omega 6s to omega 3s in the American diet is believed to be as high as 14:1 (14 grams of omega 6s for every 1 gram of omega 3s); a ratio of no more than 3:1 (3 grams of omega 6s for every 1 gram of omega 3) is recommended. (See "ConsumerTips™," page 118.)

QUALITY CONCERNS

Because omega-3 fatty acids are obtained from natural sources, levels in supplements can vary, depending on the source and method of processing. Contamination is also a concern because fish can accumulate toxins, such as mercury, dioxins, and PCBs. The freshness of the oil is another consideration because rancid fish oils have an extremely unpleasant odor and may be ineffective.

Neither the FDA nor any other federal or state agency routinely tests fish or marine oil supplements for quality before sale; therefore, ConsumerLab.com independently evaluated several leading dietary supplements claiming to contain EPA or DHA and tested them for their levels of these substances. The products were also tested for contamination with mercury and for signs of decomposition.

PRODUCT TESTING

ConsumerLab.com purchased 20 omega-3 marine oil products, 19 of which were EPA/DHA combination products made from fish oils and 1 of which was a DHA-only product made from algal oil. These were tested for amounts of EPA and DHA, peroxide levels (which indicate spoilage), and contamination with mercury. (See "ConsumerLab.com's testing methods and standards," page 169.)

TEST FINDINGS

Of the 20 products tested, 6 failed to pass the review because they contained too little DHA, which ranged from 50% to 83% of the amounts stated on their labels. Of these 6 products, 2 also contained only 33% and 82%, respectively, of their labeled amounts of EPA. Interestingly, 2 products that failed made claims that their potency had been tested or verified. By providing less than claimed amounts of EPA and DHA, products may have reduced potency. For example, research has suggested that doses of about 5 grams of omega 3s a day may help protect arteries from clogging for people at high risk. Getting less than that may not provide that protection.

No product showed evidence of significant decomposition and none contained detectable levels of mercury (less than 1.5 ppb). By comparison, mercury levels in fish generally range from 10 to 1,000 ppb, depending on the fish. Possible explanations for the lack of mercury include fish species least likely to accumulate mercury may have been used; most mercury is found in fish meat, not oil; and distillation processes may have removed the contaminants.

QUALITY PRODUCTS

Listed alphabetically by name on pages 117 to 118 are the products that passed ConsumerLab.com's independent testing of EPA and DHA dietary supplements (see Omega-3 fatty acid [EPA & DHA] approved-quality products). Some products may contain other ingredients not shown.

Fish Oils

Omega-3 Fatty acid (EPA & DHA) approved-quality products

Product name (amount of fish oil, EPA, and DHA/pill)	Manufacturer (Mf) or Distributor (Dist)
EPA & DHA Combination Products	
Carlson Super Omega-3 Fish Oils (300 mg EPA and 200 mg DHA/softgel)* Laboratories, Inc.	Dist: Carlson, Division of J.R. Carlson
Dale Alexander® Omega-3 Fish Oil Concentrate (234 mg EPA and 125 mg DHA/softgel)*	Dist: Twin Laboratories, Inc.
Health From The Sun The Total EFA™ Essential Fatty Acid Dietary Supplement (72 mg EPA and 46 mg DHA/capsule)	Marketed by Health From The Sun, Div. of Arkopharma
Jarrow Formulas™ Max DHA™ Purified by Molecular Distillation 80% Omega-3 Fish Oil, 50% DHA, 20% EPA (500 mg fish oil, 100 mg EPA, and 250 mg DHA/softgel)	Mf: Jarrow Formulas, Inc.™
Member's Mark™ Omega 3 Fish Oil 1000 mg Natural Concentrate (1000 mg fish oil, 180 mg EPA, and 120 mg DHA/softgel)	Dist: SWC
Nutrilite® Omega 3 Complex Dietary Supplement »(300 mg fish oil, 65 mg EPA, and 45 mg DHA/softgel) ‡	Dist: Amway Corp. (Access Business Group International LLC [formerly Amway]
Pure Encapsulations® EPA/DHA essentials™ (1,000 mg fish oil, 300 mg EPA, and 200 mg DHA/capsule)	Mf: Pure Encapsulations, Inc.
Puritan's Pride® Inspired By Nature™ Salmon Oil 500mg (500 mg fish oil, 40 mg EPA, and 60 mg DHA/softgel)	Mf: Puritan's Pride, Inc.
Shaklee® EPA Omega-3 Fatty Acid Dietary Supplement (182 mg EPA and 78 mg DHA/capsule)	Dist: Shaklee Corp.
Solgar Omega-3 "700" EPA & DHA from Cold Water Fish (700 mg fish oil, 360 mg EPA, and 240 mg DHA/softgel)	Mf: Solgar Vitamin and Herb
Spectrum Essentials® Omega 3 Cold Processed Norwegian Fish Oil (1,000 mg fish oil, 180 mg EPA, and 120 mg DHA/capsule)	Dist: Spectrum Organic Products, Inc.

(continued)

117

Product name (amount of fish oil, EPA, and DHA/pill)	Manufacturer (Mf) or Distributor (Dist)
The Vitamin Shoppe EPA-DHA Omega-3 Fish Oil 500 (1,000 mg fish oil, 300 mg EPA, and 200 mg DHA/softgel)	Mfd. for The Vitamin Shoppe™
Trader Darwin's™ Molecularly Distilled Omega-3 Fatty Acids Dietary Supplement (1,100 mg fish oil, 300 mg EPA, and 200 mg DHA/softgel)	Dist: Trader Joe's
Vitamin World® Naturally Inspired™ EPA Natural Fish Oil 1000 mg (1,000 mg fish oil, 180 mg EPA, and 120 mg DHA/softgel)	Mf: Vitamin World, Inc.
ZonePerfect® Omega 3 Molecular Distilled Fish Oil and Vitamin E Supplement (1,000 mg fish oil, 160 mg EPA, 107 mg DHA/capsule)	Dist: ZonePerfect Nutrition Co.
DHA-Only Products	
Nature's Way® Neuromins™ Plant sourced DHA (100 mg DHA/softgel)	Dist: Nature's Way Products, Inc.

* Tested through ConsumerLab.com's Ad Hoc Testing Program (Product was tested at the manufacturer's request after the initial review was completed and released.)

‡ See "More Brand Information" page 191.

CONSUMERTIPS™ FOR BUYING AND USING

ConsumerLab.com has prepared numerous important tips about dosing, selecting, and buying fish oil — omega-3 fatty acid (EPA & DHA) supplements. This information — along with our list of approved-quality brands — provides a valuable guide for choosing appropriate products.

Products vary significantly in amounts and ratios of EPA and DHA. Versions made from menhaden and other small fish have a ratio of EPA to DHA of 1.5 — that is, a capsule claiming 1 gram (1,000 mg) of fish oil, provides 180 mg of EPA, and 120 mg of DHA, or slightly less than one-third of the fish oil comes in the form of omega 3s. However, a more concentrated product may contain twice those amounts. Some salmon oil products, for example, claim to contain more DHA than EPA and products made only from algal oil contain only DHA. A concentrated product may mean fewer capsules need to be taken.

Semisynthetic ("ester") forms of EPA and DHA are also available and are believed to be as active the natural forms. Many products also contain vitamin E or another antioxidant to prevent rancidity.

For the general population, the American Heart Association recommends at least two 3-ounce servings of fish a week. Fatty fish have the highest levels of omega-3 fatty acids, and good sources include anchovies, bluefish, carp, catfish, halibut, herring, lake trout, mackerel, pompano, salmon, striped sea bass, tuna (albacore), and whitefish, according to the U.S. Department of Agriculture (Agricultural Research Service, 2001).

A 3-ounce serving of canned tuna, contains about 2.5 grams of fat, about 30% of which is EPA (200 mg) and DHA (500 mg). Note, however, that levels of pollutants, such as mercury, tend to be higher in long-lived, larger fish having more dark meat, particularly shark, swordfish, king mackerel, and tilefish, and the FDA has advised pregnant women to avoid eating these types, because mercury may harm a fetus's developing nervous system. These fish average about 1,000 ppb of mercury—the FDA limit for human consumption. Other fish tend to have about one-tenth to one-third of this amount. Although eating a fish with 1,000 ppb of mercury isn't necessarily toxic, young children, pregnant women, and breast-feeding women shouldn't consume such fish at all, and no one should consume it on a regular basis. Fish, such as salmon and tuna (particularly white meat) are preferred sources of omega 3s and pregnant women may eat up to 12 ounces of such cooked fish per week. The Environmental Protection Agency has also advised that freshwater fish may contain more mercury than commercially caught fish and advises that "If you are pregnant or could become pregnant, are nursing a baby, or feeding a young child, limit consumption of fish caught by family and friends to one meal (about 6 ounces) of fish per week."

Eggs fortified with DHA are now available in the United States and claim to contain 150 mg of DHA in each egg, which is about the amount found in 3 ounces of salmon. Chickens producing these eggs are typically fed algal DHA. Algal DHA has been approved as a food ingredient, so foods and beverages can be fortified with DHA. Infant formulas in the United States typically don't contain EPA or DHA but have ALA as an ingredient. However, DHA is often added to formulas for premature infants. Because some formula-fed infants may not convert enough ALA to DHA, U.S. manufacturers have begun adding DHA to some formulas. In other countries, DHA is already in some regular formula as well as versions for premature infants.

The typical dosage of fish oil is 3 to 9 g/day, of which about 30% is EPA and DHA. The AHA recommends fish oil capsules for patients who have extremely high triglyceride levels (greater than 1,000 mg/dl) and haven't responded well to other treatments. In treating patients with high triglyceride levels, about 5 grams of combined EPA and DHA is recommended daily. About 3 grams of EPA and DHA is used to treat hypertension, rheumatoid arthritis, Crohn's disease, and ulcerative colitis. About 1 gram/day may protect against recurrence of a heart attack. About 9 grams/day of combined EPA and DHA, which is a fairly high dose, has been used to treat schizophrenia, and relatively high doses have also been used to treat Raynaud's phenomenon.

The recommended dosage of DHA, from either supplements or fish, for pregnant women and for breast-feeding women is 100 to 200 mg/day. Although there's no official recommended intake for omega 3s for healthy people, some experts suggest about 650 mg/day, with at least 220 mg coming from DHA and at least the same amount from EPA. The remaining 200+ mg can come from either DHA or EPA.

Fish oils are best tolerated when taken with meals and should be taken in divided doses — that is, you should divide the dose in half and take twice a day, or divide it in thirds and take three times a day.

CAUTIONS AND CONCERNS

Fish oils (DHA and EPA) are generally considered safe when taken in appropriate amounts, but be aware that the most common adverse effects are fishy smelling burps and diarrhea. Most adults can tolerate up to about 20 grams of fish oil, though most experts recommend against taking this much because it may cause bleeding. Cod liver oil isn't a good substitute for fish oil supplements because it's high in vitamins A and D, two vitamins that are toxic in excess amounts (see "Multivitamin & multiminerals," pages 33 to 53).

Hemophiliacs; individuals taking prescription blood thinners, such as warfarin (Coumadin) or heparin; and individuals expecting to undergo surgery should use fish oils only under a physician's care. Although rare, interactions may occur between EPA supplements and aspirin or other nonsteroidal anti-inflammatory drugs and herbs such as garlic and ginkgo.

Ginkgo Biloba

WHAT IT IS

Ginkgo biloba supplements come from extracts of ginkgo biloba tree leaves. The extract (GBE) used in most clinical trials contains two specific naturally occurring chemicals: flavonol glycosides and terpene lactones. Flavonol glycosides, of which there are three, may confer antioxidant activity, and terpene lactones, of which there are two categories, may be responsible for ginkgo's dilatory effect on blood vessels as well as its blood-thinning properties. For gingko biloba supplements to be effective, these chemicals must be present in a specific quantity of clinical quality GBE. (The chemicals can, therefore, represent a standard for assessing ginkgo products). Many GBE products claim to be standardized or manufactured to contain specific amounts of flavonol glycosides or terpene lactones.

WHAT IT DOES

Ginkgo biloba is widely used for increasing cognitive function in elderly people with dementia or Alzheimer's disease, for increasing blood flow to the legs, as well as for treating depression, asthma, and tinnitus (ringing in the ear) resulting from circulation problems. At least one study suggests gingko may also be useful for treating sexual dysfunction caused by antidepressants. However, in treating dementia, it isn't clear whether ginkgo biloba delays deterioration, as some studies have suggested, or temporarily improves symptoms.

How does ginkgo biloba work? The exact mechanism is uncertain, but it has both antioxidant and anti-inflammatory properties, which may increase blood flow to the brain. It may also strengthen capillaries in the brain or prevent the oxidation of cell membranes, say researchers. Though ginkgo may be helpful as a treatment for dementia and Alzheimer's, there's no evidence that it can prevent or reverse the decline in memory and cognitive function that commonly occurs with age. Ginkgo biloba extract is well tolerated with few adverse effects, according to several studies.

QUALITY CONCERNS
Because no government agency is responsible for routinely testing ginkgo biloba supplements for their contents or quality, ConsumerLab.com independently evaluated several leading gingko biloba products to determine whether they contained GBE of the quality most similar to that used in clinical trials. The products were also tested to determine whether they contained the amounts of appropriate plant chemicals indicated on their labels.

PRODUCT TESTING
ConsumerLab.com purchased 30 leading brands of ginkgo biloba and tested them for their amounts of flavonol glycosides and terpene lactones. (See "ConsumerLab.com's testing methods and standards," page 169.)

TEST FINDINGS
Nearly one-quarter of the brands tested didn't contain the expected levels of chemical marker compounds for GBE. Among these, all had less-than-adequate levels of one or more terpene lactones, and 3 also lacked adequate levels of one or more flavone glycosides. Even though they didn't pass testing, all had labels claiming standardization for flavone glycosides; most indicated they'd been standardized for terpene lactones as well. Some of the products met their label claims for total terpene lactones or total flavone glycosides but did not contain the right amounts of specific terpene lactones or flavone glycosides to pass the review.

Ginkgo biloba approved-quality products

Product name (concentration of extract/pill)	Manufacturer (Mf) or distributor (Dist)
Acuity Plus, Ginkgo Biloba, (40 mg/caplet)	Mf: Shaklee
Centrum Herbals, Standardized Ginkgo Biloba Natural Dietary Supplement, (60 mg/capsule)	Mf: Whitehall-Robins Healthcare
Country Life, Herbal Formula, Ginkgo Biloba Extract (60 mg/capsule)	Mf: Country Life
CVS, Premium Quality Herbs, Ginkgo Biloba Standardized Extract, (120 mg/caplet)	Dist: CVS
Enzymatic Therapy, Ginkgo Biloba 24% (40 mg/capsule)*	Mf: Enzymatic Therapy
Ginkai, Ginkgo Biloba (50 mg/tablet)	Mf: Lichtwer Pharma
Ginkgo Biloba and DHA (53.3 mg/softgel)* ‡	Mf: Nutrilite (Access Business Group International LLC [formerly Amway])
Ginkgo Biloba Plus with Aged Garlic Extract, Ginkgo Biloba (40 mg/capsule)	Mf: Wakunaga of America
Ginkgo-go, Triple Strength Formula, Ginkgo Biloba (120 mg/caplet)	Mf: Wakunaga Consumer Products
Ginkgold, Ginkgo Biloba (60 mg/tablet)	Mf: Nature's Way
Ginkgolidin, Ginkgo Biloba Standardized Extract (40 mg/capsule)*	Mf: PhytoPharmica
Ginkoba, Mental Performance Dietary Supplement, Ginkgo Biloba (40 mg/tablet)	Mf: Pharmaton Natural Health Products
GNC, Natural Brand (50 mg/tablet)	Mf: GNC
MotherNature.com, Standardized Ginkgo Biloba Extract (60 mg/capsule)	Mfd. for MotherNature.com
Natrol, Ginkgo Biloba (60 mg/capsule)	Mf: Natrol, Inc
Nature Made Herbs, Ginkgo Biloba (40 mg/softgel) ‡	Mf: Nature Made Nutritional Products
Nature's Bounty, Herbal Harvest, Ginkgo Biloba (30 mg/tablet)	Mf: Nature's Bounty
Nature's Resource, Premium Herb, Extra Strength, Ginkgo Biloba (60 mg/capsule)‡	Dist: N.R. Products
NOW Ginkgo Biloba 24% Standard Extract (60 mg/capsule)*	Mf: NOW Foods

Product name (concentration of extract/pill)	Manufacturer (Mf) or distributor (Dist)
One-A-Day, Memory and Concentration, Ginkgo Biloba (60 mg/tablet)	Mf: Bayer
Puritans' Pride, Inspired by Nature, Ginkgo Biloba Standardized Extract (60 mg/tablet)	Mf: NBTY
Quanterra, Mental Sharpness, Ginkgo Biloba (60 mg/tablet)	Mf: Warner-Lambert
Spring Valley, Ginkgo Biloba Dietary Supplement, Standardized Extract (40 mg/tablet)	Mf: Leiner Health Products Inc. Dist: Walmart
Sundown Herbals, Ginkgo Biloba, For Mental Alertness (20 mg/capsule)	Dist: Sundown Vitamins
Thompson, Ginkgo Biloba (60 mg/capsule)	Mf: Thompson Nutritional Products
Walgreens, Ginkgo Biloba Standardized Extract (60 mg/tablet)	Dist: Walgreens
Your Life, Ginkgo Biloba Standardized Herbal Extract (60 mg/caplet)	Mf: Leiner Health Products Inc.

* Tested through ConsumerLab.com's Ad Hoc Testing Program (Product was tested at the manufacturer's request after the initial review was completed and released.)
‡ See "More information about brands" page 191.
Copyright ConsumerLab.com, LLC, 2000, 2001, 2002, 2003. All rights reserved. Not to be reproduced, excerpted, or cited without written permission from ConsumerLab.com LLC.

QUALITY PRODUCTS

Listed alphabetically above by name are the products that passed ConsumerLab.com's independent testing of gingko biloba dietary supplements (see Ginkgo biloba approved-quality products).

CONSUMERTIPS™ FOR BUYING AND USING

ConsumerLab.com has prepared numerous important tips about dosing, selecting, and buying ginkgo biloba supplements. This information — along with our list of approved-quality brands — provides a valuable guide for choosing appropriate products.

The ideal composition of GBE for specific medical conditions isn't known. However, consumers seeking products similar to those used in clinical studies should look for GBE standardized for the specific compounds used in the study. Standardized compounds may, for example, be listed as 24% flavone glycosides and 6% terpene lactones, or they may be listed in terms of milligrams for a 40-mg pill—for example, 9.6 mg of flavone glycosides and 2.4 mg of terpene lactones. Unfortunately, labels aren't always accurate.

A daily dose of 120 mg of GBE (taken in doses of 40 mg or 60 mg over the course of the day, not in a single dose) is generally recommended. It may take several weeks for results to be apparent. European health authorities recommend a daily dose of up to 240 mg/day for more severe cases of dementia.

CAUTIONS AND CONCERNS

GBE is generally considered safe when taken in appropriate amounts, but be aware that ginkgo can have a blood-thinning effect, so check with your physician before taking it along with other blood-thinning drugs, such as warfarin (Coumadin) or aspirin. Also, know that ginkgo may cause nervousness, headache, and stomachache in some people.

Ginseng

WHAT IT IS

Ginseng is the dried root of one of several species of the Araliaceae family of herbs. The most commonly used type is Asian ginseng (Panax ginseng C.A., Meyer), often sold as Panax, Chinese, or Korean ginseng. Closely related to Asian ginseng is American ginseng (Panax quinquefolius L.), which is sometimes preferred for its milder effects. Siberian ginseng, also called eleuthero (Eleutherococcus senticosus Rupr ex Maxim), isn't as closely related to the other two and contains a series of unrelated compounds. Siberian ginseng is also considered weaker in action and is a less expensive ingredient. Ginseng-containing dietary supplements are typically made from a powder or extract of ginseng root.

WHAT IT DOES

Ginseng is widely used in the United States to improve overall energy and vitality, particularly during times of fatigue or stress. Other reported uses of ginseng include normalizing blood sugar levels in people with diabetes, stimulating immune function, and treating male impotence. Ginseng has been shown to allow cells to readily use stored sugar and to enable red blood cells to carry oxygen. However, the clinical evidence for ginseng's effectiveness has been mixed. Plant chemicals called ginsenosides are believed to play a role in ginseng's activity. They are considered "marker" compounds for ginseng—that is, their presence (or absence) and their chemical profiles can indicate the type and quality of ginseng in a product.

QUALITY CONCERNS

Pesticide and heavy-metal contamination are safety concerns in some botanical products. For example, the pesticide pentachloronitrobenzene (known as quintozene or PCNB), a possible carcinogen that may also be toxic to the liver and kidneys and may impair oxygen transport in the blood, has been reported in samples of ginseng. Other pesticides of concern are hexachlorobenzene and lindane, which are possible carcinogens. Hexachlorobenzene has been banned from most food-crop use throughout the world and quinitozene and lindane generally aren't allowed for use on U.S. food crops.

Because no government agency is responsible for routinely testing ginseng supplements for their contents or quality, ConsumerLab.com independently evaluated several leading ginseng products to determine whether they contained the type and amount of ginseng stated on their labels. The products were also tested for contamination with pesticides and heavy metals.

PRODUCT TESTING

ConsumerLab.com purchased 22 brands of Asian and American ginseng products and tested them for total ginsenosides and contamination with heavy metals and pesticides. (See "ConsumerLab.com's testing methods and standards," page 169.)

TEST FINDINGS

Of the 22 products tested, 17 were Asian (labeled as Panax ginseng, Asian ginseng, Chinese ginseng, or Korean ginseng), 4 were American ginseng, and 1 was a mixture of Asian, American, and Siberian ginseng. One American ginseng product made from root powder was immediately eliminated from testing because it was labeled to contain only 0.589% ginsenosides, which is below the 2% minimum for American ginseng root powder required to pass ConsumerLab.com's testing.

Only 9 products tested met all criteria for ginseng quality and purity. Each passing product was also found to meet California's stringent standard for lead levels.

Of the 21 products that were tested, 12 didn't pass in one or more of the following criteria: 8 products contained unacceptable levels of both quintozene and hexachlorobenzene, 2 products had pesticide levels

Ginseng approved-quality products

Product name (type of ginseng) (labeled amount, ginsenoside concentration, if given)	Manufacturer (Mf) and/or distributor (Dist)
Celestial Seasonings Ginseng (Asian) (100 mg/capsule, 7% ginsenosides).	Mf: Celestial Seasonings, Inc
Centrum Herbals Ginseng (Asian) (100 mg/capsule, 7% ginsenosides)	Dist: Whitehall-Robins Healthcare
Ginsana (Asian) (100 mg softgel, 4% ginsenosides)	Dist: Pharmaton Natural Health Products
NaturaLife Ultra Active Ginseng (Korean) (150 mg/softgel, 5% ginsenosides)	Dist: NaturaLife Corp.
Nature Made Chinese Red Panax Ginseng (250 mg/softgel)	Dist: Nature Made Nutritional Products
One A Day Energy Formula (American) (200 mg/tablet)	Dist: Bayer Corp.
PharmAssure Standardized Korean Ginseng (500 mg/capsule, 4% ginsenosides)	Dist: PharmAssure
Root to Health American Ginseng (500 mg/capsule)	Dist: Hsu's Ginseng Enterprises, Inc.
Walgreens Finest Gin-Zing Concentrate (Asian) (100 mg/softgel)	Dist: Walgreen Co.

more than 20 times the allowed amount, 2 products contained lead above the acceptable level (3 mcg/day), and 7 products had less than the required concentration of ginsenosides. No product, however, surpassed the limit for the pesticide lindane or was found to contain significant levels of arsenic or cadmium.

Interestingly, all 8 products that contained lead or pesticides were labeled as containing Korean ginseng. In fact, only 2 of the 12 products containing Korean ginseng passed. Among the 8 Korean ginseng products contaminated with pesticides, 3 also had low ginsenoside levels and 2 others had high levels of lead. Two Korean ginseng products failed solely on low ginsenoside levels.

QUALITY PRODUCTS

Listed alphabetically by name on page 129 are products that passed ConsumerLab.com's independent testing of ginseng (see Ginseng approved-quality products).

CONSUMERTIPS™ FOR BUYING AND USING

ConsumerLab.com has prepared numerous important tips about dosing, selecting, and buying ginseng supplements. This information — along with our list of approved-quality brands — provides a valuable guide for choosing appropriate products.

Product labels should ideally indicate the type of ginseng, the form (powder or extract), the percent concentration of ginsenosides, and the amount of ginseng per tablet in milligrams (mg) or grams. This information should also be considered when comparing the cost of products. For example, among the products evaluated, the labeled amount of ginseng root extract ranged from 100 to 200 mg/tablet, whereas the labeled amount of ginseng root powder ranged from 150 to 500 mg/tablet. Unfortunately, the labels may be inaccurate. For example, among the 15 products stating ginsenoside concentrations on their labels, only 10 met or exceeded these claims.

Generally recommended daily doses of ginseng are 200 mg of a standardized extract (minimum of 3% total ginsenosides for Asian ginseng and minimum of 4% total ginsenosides for American ginseng, although some products may contain higher levels) taken as 100 mg twice daily, or 1,000 to 2,000 mg (1 to 2 grams) of root powder per day. Effects may take a few days before onset.

CAUTIONS AND CONCERNS

Ginseng is generally safe when taken in appropriate amounts, but be aware that high doses may cause overstimulation and insomnia, which can be exacerbated by excessive caffeine intake. The herb may also cause hypertension, and with long-term use, hypoglycemia and menstrual abnormalities.

Ginseng may interact with estrogens and blood thinners such as warfarin (Coumadin).

The safety of ginseng hasn't been well evaluated during pregnancy or breast-feeding; therefore, using ginseng during those times isn't recommended.

Glucosamine & chondroitin

WHAT IT IS

Glucosamine and chondroitin sulfate both occur naturally in the body. The glucosamine used in supplements is derived from the shells of crabs, and chondroitin typically comes from cow cartilage.

WHAT IT DOES

Glucosamine and chondroitin sulfate supplements are used to slow the progression of osteoarthritis — the deterioration of cartilage between joint bones — and to reduce the associated pain. Glucosamine is thought to promote the formation and repair of cartilage. Chondroitin is believed to promote water retention and elasticity in cartilage and inhibit enzymes that break down cartilage.

QUALITY CONCERNS

Chondroitin is an expensive material, so experts have been concerned about the quality and quantity of the ingredient in supplements. Because chondroitin typically comes from cow cartilage, an additional concern has been whether the products may be contaminated with bovine spongiform encephalitis, the causative agent (a "prion") of Mad Cow Disease. The risk, however, seems to be miniscule for several reasons: First, the chondroitin would have to come from an infected cow, of which none have been reported in the United States. However, imports of chondroitin haven't received the same scrutiny as meat products. Second, the prion is known to exist only in very low levels in cartilage;

it's most abundant in nervous and glandular tissue. Third, some manufacturers have stated that the process used to make chondroitin supplements should inactivate the prion—although this hasn't been shown conclusively. Unfortunately, there's no simple way to test for BSE prion contamination in supplements, so products in this review weren't evaluated for contamination.

Because no government agency is responsible for routinely testing glucosamine and condroitin supplements for their contents or quality, ConsumerLab.com independently evaluated several leading glucosamine and condroitin products to determine whether they contained the amounts of glucosamine and condroitin stated on their labels.

PRODUCT TESTING

ConsumerLab.com purchased 25 brands of glucosamine, chondroitin and combined glucosamine-chondroitin products and tested them for quality. Of the 25 brands tested, 10 were labeled glucosamine only, 2 were labeled chondroitin only, and 13 were a combination of the two. (See "ConsumerLab.com's testing methods and standards," page 169.)

TEST FINDINGS

Overall, nearly one-third of the 25 products didn't pass testing. Among glucosamine-chondroitin combination products, almost half (6 out of 13) didn't pass because of low chondroitin levels. Similarly, 2 chondroitin-only products didn't pass. However, all 10 glucosamine-only products passed. One possible explanation for the low pass rate for chondroitin-containing products is economics—chondroitin costs manufacturers about four times as much as glucosamine.

Note: ConsumerLab.com removed 1 originally approved glucosamine-chondroitin combination product from its list of passing products. Why? The product, based on information on its "Supplement Facts" panel, exceeded the new tolerable upper level intake (UL) for manganese set by the National Academies' Institute of Medicine. Significant levels of manganese may be found in some multivitamin and multimineral supplements and should also be considered when calculating total daily intake of manganese. (See "Manganese" in "Multivitamins & multiminerals," page 51.)

QUALITY PRODUCTS

Listed alphabetically by name on pages 134 to 135 are the products that passed ConsumerLab.com's independent testing of glucosamine and chondroitin dietary supplements (see Glucosamine and chondroitin approved-quality products).

CONSUMERTIPS™ FOR BUYING AND USING

ConsumerLab.com has prepared numerous important tips about dosing, selecting, and buying glucosamine and chondroitin supplements. This information — along with our list of approved-quality brands — provides a valuable guide for choosing appropriate products.

Glucosamine supplements are sold in many forms, including glucosamine sulfate–2KCl (potassium chloride), glucosamine sulfate, glucosamine hydrochloride (HCl), and N-acetylglucosamine (NAG), and may also contain a sodium chloride salt. However, there's no conclusive evidence that one form is better than another. Chondroitin is typically sold as chondroitin sulfate, the form used in most studies.

Consumers should check product labels to be sure products provide 1,000 mg of "free" glucosamine, approximately the amount found in 1,700 mg of glucosamine sulfate–2KCl or 1,270 mg of glucosamine sulfate or 1,200 mg of glucosamine HCl or 1,230 mg of NAG. People limiting their salt intake should be aware that many products made with sulfate have salt added to help stabilize the ingredients. About 1,200 mg of chondroitin sulfate is recommended per day.

Both glucosamine and chondroitin should be taken in divided doses throughout the day (that is, 500 mg of glucosamine HCl and 400 mg of chondroitin sulfate three times per day). Because the amount of glucosamine or chondroitin per pill varies across products, the number of pills needed daily varies and this should be considered when comparing the costs of products.

Some glucosamine-chondroitin products may contain manganese (possibly to aid bone formation). However, the manganese levels in such products typically exceed the recommended intake and, in many cases, are also in excess of the UL. The recommended intake is 2.3 mg/day for men and 1.8 mg/day for women — an amount similar to that consumed in the typical American diet.

Glucosamine & chondroitin approved-quality products

Product name (concentration of main ingredient(s)/pill	Manufacturer (Mf) or Distributor (Dist)
Glucosamine & Chondroitin Sulfate Combination Products	
ArthxDS™ Glucosamine Chondroitin (500 mg glucosamine HCl and 400 mg chondroitin sulfate/capsule)*	Dist: Medtech (Mfd. by PECOS Pharmaceuticals)
ArthxDS™ Once Per Day Time Release Formula Glucosamine 1500 mg Chondroitin 1200 mg (750 mg glucosamine HCl and 600 mg chondroitin sulfate/caplet)*	Dist: Medtech (Mfd. by PECOS Pharmaceuticals)
Double Strength Cosamin®DS (500 mg glucosamine HCl, 400 mg chondroitin sulfate, and 5 mg manganese/capsule)* ‡	Mf: Nutramax Laboratories, Inc.
Glucosamine/Chondroitin Double Strength (500 mg glucosamine HCl and 400 mg chondroitin/capsule)	Dist: Walgreens
Maximum Strength Flex-A-Min® Glucosamine, Chondroitin, MSM (500 mg glucosamine sulfate–2KCl and 400 mg chondroitin/tablet)*	Mf and Dist: Arthritis Research Corp.
Maximum Strength Glucosamine/Chondroitin (500 mg glucosamine HCl and 400 mg chondroitin/tablet)	Dist: CVS
Move Free Joint Support Formula tablets (500 mg glucosamine sulfate, glucosamine HCl, N-acetylglucosamine, and 400 mg chondroitin/tablet)	Dist: Schiff
Nature's Bounty Chondroitin Complex with Glucosamine (250 mg glucosamine HCl and 200 mg chondroitin/capsule)	Mf: Nature's Bounty
Osteo-Bi-Flex Glucosamine/Chondroitin (250 mg glucosamine HCl and 200 mg chondroitin/tablet)	Mfd for Dist: Sundown
Spring Valley Glucosamine/Chondroitin Max. Strength (500 mg glucosamine HCl and 400 mg chondroitin/tablet)	Wal-Mart/Mf: Park-Taft Laboratories
Triple FlexTMMaximum Strength Glucosamine Chondroitin Plus MSM Supplement (500 mg glucosamine HCl and 400 mg chondroitin sulfate/tablet)* ‡	Dist: Nature Made

Glucosamine & chondroitin

Glucosamine-Only Products

Aflexa Glucosamine (sulfate) (340 mg/tablet)*	Dist: McNeil Consumer Healthcare, Inc.
Enzymatic Therapy GS-500, Glucosamine Sulfate (500 mg/capsule)*	Mfd. by Enzymatic Therapy
Fields of Nature Glucosamine Sulfate, Natural Joint Nutrient (500 mg capsules)	Dist: Fields of Nature
GNC Glucosamine (sulfate) (600 mg/capsule)	Dist: GNC
Natrol Glucosamine Complex—sulfate, HCl, and N-acetyl (500 mg/capsule)	Mfd. by Natrol
Nature Made® Glucosamine (sulfate and HCl) (500 mg/tablet) ‡	Dist: Nature Made
Nature Made® Joint Action™, (500 mg glucosamine HCl/tablet)* ‡	Dist: Nature Made
Now Glucosamine Sulfate 750 mg Complex (750 mg glucosamine sulfate–2KCl/capsule)*	Dist: Now Foods
Nutrilite Glucosamine HCl with Boswellia (375 mg/caplet) ‡	Dist: Access Business Group International LLC
One A Day Joint Health (with Glucosamine and Vitamins C & E) (500 mg glucosamine sulfate/tablet)*	Dist: Bayer
OsteoJoint Triple Formula for Healthy Joints (500 mg glucosamine sulfate/caplet)	Dist: Your Life
Osteokinetics (467 mg glucosamine HCl /capsule)	Dist: Shaklee (Formulas)
PhytoPharmica Glucosamine Sulfate (500 mg/capsule)*	Mf: PhytoPharmica
Puritans' Pride Glucosamine Sulfate (1,000 mg/capsule)	Mf: Puritans' Pride
Spring Valley Glucosamine Complex— sulfate and HCl (500 mg/tablet)	Wal-Mart/Mf: Leiner Health Products

Chondroitin Sulfate–Only Products

NOW Chondroitin Sulfate (600 mg/capsule)*	Dist: Now Foods

* Tested through ConsumerLab.com's Ad Hoc Testing Program (Product was tested at the manufacturer's request after the initial review was completed and released.)

‡ See "More Brand Information," page 191.

Beneficial effects from these products may take anywhere from several weeks to 4 months, and the products aren't likely to help those with severe osteoarthritis — where cartilage has worn down so much that bones rub against bones. Losing weight and switching from high-impact to low-impact sports are also advised for people with osteoarthritis.

CAUTIONS AND CONCERNS

Glucosamine and chondroitin, taken in appropriate amounts, are generally considered safe for healthy people not taking other medications, but be aware that, in a some individuals, glucosamine can cause gastrointestinal discomfort, drowsiness, skin reactions, and headache and chondroitin can occasionally cause stomach upset.

Glucosamine is an amino sugar, so it may also affect blood sugar levels. Consequently, people with diabetes should check their blood sugar levels frequently when taking this supplement, and anyone noticing an increased blood sugar level should alert his physician and consider discontinuing use of the product. Because the glucosamine in supplements is commonly derived from crab shells, people allergic to shellfish may experience an allergic reaction to these products.

Chondroitin is similar in structure to the blood-thinning drug heparin, so use of chondroitin with blood-thinning drugs or daily aspirin therapy may cause bleeding in some people.

MSM

WHAT IT IS

Methylsulfonylmethane (MSM), also known as dimethyl sulfone (DMSO$_2$), is a sulfur-containing compound occurring naturally in plants and animals, although its natural biological role is unknown. As a veterinary medicine, MSM is used to treat muscle and tendon soreness and inflammation in horses.

WHAT IT DOES

As a dietary supplement, MSM is used primarily for treating pain associated with osteoarthritis and has been proposed for treating other conditions including rheumatoid arthritis, inflammation of the bladder wall (interstitial cystitis), snoring, muscle spasm, and cancer. All of these uses, including those for arthritis, are based on limited research, so its effectiveness hasn't been well established. Many additional claims are found on MSM products, including skin-softening and nail-strengthening effects, but none of these are well supported by research.

The mechanism by which MSM may work isn't well understood, although it's known to contribute sulfur to the body, which can then be used to synthesize certain amino acids (building blocks for proteins), and it can act as an antioxidant. MSM is chemically related to DMSO (dimethyl sulfoxide), which has been used in ways similar to MSM. Unlike MSM, however, DMSO is a chemical solvent. DMSO was found to cause a range of adverse reactions and is no longer approved as a supplement. It still has limited use, however, for those under medical supervision.

QUALITY CONCERNS

Because no government agency is responsible for routinely testing MSM supplements for their contents or quality, ConsumerLab.com independently evaluated several leading MSM products to determine whether they contained the amounts of MSM stated on their labels. The products were also tested for DMSO contamination. Although not thought to be a health risk in small amounts, DMSO in products indicates poor-quality manufacturing.

PRODUCT TESTING

ConsumerLab.com purchased 17 MSM dietary supplements, several of which also contained other ingredients, such as glucosamine, chondroitin, or vitamin C. The products were tested for their labeled amounts of MSM and for contamination with DMSO. (See "ConsumerLab.com's testing methods and standards," page 169.)

TEST FINDINGS

Of the 17 products tested, 2 failed testing because they contained only 85% and 88% of their labeled amounts of MSM; 1 product that failed had a small amount (0.05% by weight) of DMSO. All other products had less than this amount or no detectable DMSO.

QUALITY PRODUCTS

Listed alphabetically here by name are the products that passed ConsumerLab.com's independent testing of MSM dietary supplements (see MSM approved-quality products). Note: Some of these products may also be listed among those passing ConsumerLab.com's glucosamine and chondroitin product review. However, any MSM combination product that previously failed another ConsumerLab.com product review was ineligible for evaluation in the MSM review.

CONSUMERTIPS™ FOR BUYING AND USING

ConsumerLab.com has prepared numerous important tips about dosing, selecting, and buying MSM supplements. This information — along with our list of approved-quality brands — provides a valuable guide for choosing appropriate products.

High-quality MSM is an odorless white crystalline powder. When

MSM approved-quality supplements

Product name (amount/pill, pill type)	Manufacturer (Mf) or distributor (Dist)
Action Labs® Muscle and Joint Formula Super MSM Plus Glucosamine™ Methylsulfonylmethane with NutraFlora® (600 mg per tablet)	Mf: Nutraceutical Corp.
Cowboy Smart MSM (1,000 mg/tablet)	Dist: John Ewing Comp.
CVS MSM 1000 mg (1,000/tablet)	Dist: CVS Pharmacy, Inc.
Doctor's Best Synergistic Glucosamine/MSM Formula Dietary Supplement, Sodium Free (500 mg/capsule)	Dist: Doctor's Best, Inc.
Jarrow Formulas™ MSM 1000 Methyl-Sulfonyl-Methane (1,000 mg/tablet)	Dist: Jarrow Formulas, Inc.
Maximum Strength Flex-A-Min® Glucosamine Chondroitin MSM (167 mg/tablet)	Mf: Arthritis Research Corp.
Methylsulfonylmethane with NutraFlora® (600 mg/tablet)	Mf: Nutraceutical Corp. for Action Labs, Inc.
Natural Balance® MSM Methylsulfonylmethane (1,000 mg/tablet)	Dist: Natural Balance, Inc.
Nature's Bounty Maximum Strength Glucosamine MSM Complex (333 mg/tablet)	Mf: Nature's Bounty, Inc.
Nature's Bounty MSM Methylsulfonylmethane 750 mg (750 mg/per capsule)	Mf: Nature's Bounty, Inc.
Nature's Plus Advanced Therapeutic MSM Rx-Wellness (with Vitamin C) (1,000 mg/tablet)	Mf: Natural Organics Laboratories, Inc.
NOW MSM Lignisul MSM® 1000 mg (1,000 mg/capsule)	Dist: NOW FOODS
PlanetRx MSM (Methylsulfonylmethane) OptiMSM 1000 mg (1,000 mg/tablet)	Dist: PlanetRx.com, Inc.
Spring Valley MSM Glucosamine (250 mg/capsule)	Mf: Nature's Bounty, Inc.
Spring Valley MSM Methylsulfonylmethane 500 mg (500 mg/capsule)	Mf: Nature's Bounty, Inc.
Triple Flex™ Maximum Strength Glucosamine Chondroitin Plus MSM Supplement (125 mg/tablet)*‡	Dist: Nature Made
Vitamin World® Naturally Inspired™ MSM 1500 mg (1,500 mg/tablet)	Mf: Vitamin World

* Tested through ConsumerLab.com's Ad Hoc Testing Program (Product was tested at the manufacturer's request after the initial review was completed and released.)
‡ See "More Brand Information," page 191.

improperly manufactured, it can be contaminated with DMSO, which has a faint sulfurlike or garlic smell.

Some products claim as little as 167 mg of MSM per pill; others, as much as 1,500 mg. When buying an MSM product, consider this variation, as well as the number of pills per bottle and the value of other labeled ingredients, such as glucosamine and chondroitin.

There are few well-controlled published clinical studies for MSM, so it's difficult to determine the optimal dose. The most commonly suggested daily dose is 2 grams. However, recommendations can range from 500 mg to 3 grams (1,000 mg = 1 gram). Occasionally, recommendations go as high as 8 grams/day.

CAUTIONS AND CONCERNS

MSM is generally safe when taken at recommended dosage levels, but be aware that MSM occasionally causes nausea, diarrhea, or headache.

MSM may also have an aspirin-like effect and shouldn't be used by patients already taking blood-thinning drugs, unless medically supervised.

The safety of MSM hasn't been evaluated for children or for women who are pregnant or breast-feeding, so individuals in these groups should avoid using MSM.

SAMe

WHAT IT IS

A naturally occurring compound, SAMe (also known as SAM-e, S-adenosyl-methionine, or S-adenosyl-L-methionine) is found in every cell of the body, where it's manufactured from the essential sulfur-containing amino acid methionine. Protein-rich foods are sources of this amino acid.

WHAT IT DOES

Although SAMe has many uses, it primarily functions as an antidepressant and as a treatment for osteoarthritis and associated joint pain, stiffness, and inflammation. SAMe assists the body in producing a wide range of compounds, including neurotransmitters (such as dopamine and serotonin) and cartilage components (such as glycosaminoglycans). When natural SAMe levels are low, supplements may facilitate the production of these compounds.

QUALITY CONCERNS

SAMe is an expensive ingredient, so experts have been concerned about the actual quality and quantity of SAMe in supplements. Another concern is that SAMe can break down under certain circumstances resulting in less ingredient than what's stated on the label. Furthermore, a stabilizing molecule is always added to SAMe products, often making it unclear as to the true weight of active SAMe because the weight of the inactive stabilizer may be included in the labeled amount.

Because no government agency is responsible for routinely testing SAMe supplements for their contents or quality, ConsumerLab.com independently evaluated several leading SAMe products to determine whether they possessed the SAMe amounts stated on their labels.

PRODUCT TESTING

ConsumerLab.com purchased 13 brands of SAMe and tested them for their SAMe levels. (See "ConsumerLab.com's testing methods and standards," page 169.)

TEST FINDINGS

Overall, nearly half (6 out of 13) of the products tested didn't pass testing. Among those not passing, SAMe levels were, on average, less than half the amount declared on the labels. For 1 product, the amount of SAMe was below detectable levels (less than 5% of the labeled amount). Also, 3 products didn't pass testing because of inaccurate labeling—for example, 1 product's label claimed 200 mg of SAMe per tablet, but this weight actually included the weight of the stabilizing compound (the product really contained only about 100 mg of free SAMe per tablet).

QUALITY PRODUCTS

Listed alphabetically here by name are the products that passed ConsumerLab.com's independent testing of SAMe dietary supplements (see SAMe approved-quality products).

CONSUMERTIPS™ FOR BUYING AND USING

ConsumerLab.com has prepared numerous important tips about dosing, selecting, and buying SAMe supplements. This information — along with our list of approved-quality brands — provides a valuable guide for choosing appropriate products.

SAMe is sold with added compounds for stabilizing the SAMe molecule and preventing degradation. These compounds include tosylate, disulfate tosylate, disulfate ditosylate, and 1,4-butanedisulfonate (Actimet), and they're usually written immediately after SAMe's chemical name. Typically, the compounds weigh as much as the SAMe molecule itself. Consequently, a tablet containing 200 mg of S-adenosyl-methionine disulfate tosylate contains only 100 mg of SAMe. Most, but not all labels, make this clear.

An appropriate dosage of SAMe should exclude the stabilizing compound. In the products evaluated, the labeled amount of SAMe ranged from 100 to 200 mg/tablet.

Enteric-coated products, which aren't likely to break down in the

SAMe approved-quality products

Product name, concentration/pill (form of SAMe)	Manufacturer (Mf) or distributor (Dist)
GNC SAMe, 100 mg (Actimet® - 1,4-butanedisulfonate)	Dist: GNC
Natrol SAMe, 200 mg (disulfate ditosylate)	Dist: Natrol
Nature Made® Joint ActionTM 200 mg (1,4-butanedisolfonate)* ‡	Dist: Nature Made
Nature Made® SAM-e, 200 mg (1,4-butanedisulfonate)	Dist: Nature Made
Nature Made® SAM-e, 200 mg (tosylate disulfate)* ‡	Dist: Nature Made
NutraLife SAMe, 200 mg (tosylate disulfate)*	Dist: NutraLife Health Products
Puritan's Pride Inspired by Nature SAM-e, 200 mg (form not indicated)	Mfd for Puritan's Pride
Source Naturals SAMe, 200 mg (disulfate tosylate)	Dist: Source Naturals
The Vitamin Shoppe SAMe, 200 mg (1,4-butanedisulfonate, disulphate [sic] tosylate)	Dist: The Vitamin Shoppe
Twinlab SAM-e, 200 mg (tosylate)	Dist: Twin Laboratories

* Tested through ConsumerLab.com's Ad Hoc Testing Program (Product was tested at the manufacturer's request after the initial review was completed and released.)

‡ See "More Brand Information," page 191.

stomach, are available, and consumers should look for them, to prevent possible nausea and stomach upset. SAMe is absorbed from the intestine.

Recommended daily doses of SAMe range from 200 to 800 mg, depending on the condition, its severity, and course of treatment. Most experts recommend starting with a dose of 200 to 400 mg SAMe for the first day of therapy and increasing thereafter. These daily amounts should be taken in divided doses, such as 200 mg twice a day for a 400-mg total daily dose or 200 mg four times a day for an 800-mg total daily dose. After starting SAMe supplementation, improvements may take anywhere from a few days to 5 weeks to become noticeable.

Losing weight and switching from high-impact to low-impact sports are also recommended for people with osteoarthritis.

CAUTIONS AND CONCERNS
SAMe is generally considered safe when taken in appropriate doses, but be aware that it may occasionally cause nausea and stomach upset, adverse effects that can be reduced by taking enteric-coated products, reducing the SAMe dosage, or taking SAMe with meals.

Individuals with bipolar (manic/depressive) disorder should know that SAMe could trigger a manic phase. Also, SAMe products aren't likely to help severe osteoarthritis where cartilage has worn down so much that bones rub against bones.

Saw palmetto

WHAT IT IS

Saw palmetto is a type of palm tree, also known as the dwarf palm. Its primary medicinal value lies in the oily compounds found in its berries. Most dietary supplements are a berry extract, although crushed berry products are also available.

WHAT IT DOES

Saw palmetto, which inhibits the action of testosterone, is used primarily to improve urinary flow and reduce urinary frequency and urgency in men with prostate enlargement (benign prostatic hyperplasia). Saw palmetto has also been used to treat bladder inflammation (cystitis), chronic bronchitis, laryngitis, asthma-associated nasal inflammation, and other conditions.

Fatty acids and sterols are saw palmetto's main components. It may be that the fatty acids are responsible for saw palmetto's testosterone-inhibiting effects. The action of the sterols isn't well understood, although the sterols are present in other herbs (Pygeum bark, stinging nettle root, and pumpkin seed extract) used for treating prostate conditions. To be effective, at least 85% of the weight of clinical-quality saw palmetto products should come from specific fatty acids and sterols.

QUALITY CONCERNS

Growing, harvesting, and processing conditions affect the types and amounts of fatty acids and sterols in saw palmetto berries and extracts.

The concern: Do saw palmetto products actually contain the ingredients and amounts specified on their labels?

Because no government agency is responsible for routinely testing saw palmetto supplements for their contents or quality, ConsumerLab.com independently evaluated several leading saw palmetto products to determine whether they contained the types of fatty acids and sterols used in published clinical trials.

PRODUCT TESTING

ConsumerLab.com purchased 27 leading brands of saw palmetto and tested them for the quality and quantity of the main ingredient. (See "ConsumerLab.com's testing methods and standards," page 169.)

TEST FINDINGS

Of the 27 leading brands of saw palmetto purchased, 5 were immediately eliminated from testing because their labels claimed that they had been standardized to contain less than 85% fatty acids — specifically, 20% to 25%, 40%, 45%, 80%, and 80% fatty acids. A sixth product was eliminated because it had incomplete labeling, making it impossible to determine the amount of saw palmetto per serving.

Among the 21 remaining products tested, 4 didn't contain the minimum amounts of the specific fatty acids or sterols used in published clinical trials. Of the 4, all had low fatty acid levels, 1 had low sterol levels, and another had no detectable level of saw palmetto sterols.

Of the 17 products that passed, most contained additional oils generally identified as part of a "prostate formula." These combinations haven't been clinically tested and may not have additional benefit. Two passing products appeared to contain exclusively the saw palmetto extract similar to that used in most clinical trials.

QUALITY PRODUCTS

Listed alphabetically by name on pages 147 to 148 are the products that passed ConsumerLab.com's independent testing of saw palmetto dietary supplements (see Saw palmetto approved-quality products).

Saw palmetto approved-quality products

Product name (concentration/pill)	Manufacturer (Mf) or distributor (Dist)
Celestial Seasonings Prostate Health Ultimate Blend with Saw Palmetto, Berry and Standardized Extract, (106.66 mg/capsule)	Mf: Celestial Seasonings, Inc.
Centrum Herbals Saw Palmetto, Standardized Extract (160 mg/softgel)	Dist: Whitehall-Robins Healthcare
CVS Premium Quality Herbs Saw Palmetto Standardized Extract (160 mg/softgel)	Dist: CVS
GNC Herbal Plus Standardized Saw Palmetto (Extract) (160 mg/softgel)	Dist: General Nutrition (Extract)Corp.
MotherNature.com Standardized Saw Palmetto Extract (160 mg/softgel)	Mfd. for MotherNature.com
Natrol Saw Palmetto (Standardized Extract) (160 mg/softgel)	Dist: Natrol, Inc.
Nature's Way Standardized Saw Palmetto Extract (160 mg/softgel)	Dist: Nature's Way Products Inc.
Nutrilite Saw Palmetto (Standardized Extract) and Nettle Root (106 mg/softgel)	Dist: Access Business Group International, LLC.
One-A-Day Prostate Health, Saw Palmetto Standardized Extract (160 mg/softgel)	Dist: Bayer Corporation
PharmAssure Standardized (Extract) Saw Palmetto (160 mg/softgel)	Dist: PharmAssure, Inc.
Propalmex, Saw Palmetto Standardized Extract (160 mg/softgel)	Dist: Chattem, Inc.
ProstaPro, Saw Palmetto Berry Extract, Standardized Extract (160 mg/softgel capsule)*	Mfd. for PhytoPharmica
Puritans' Pride Saw Palmetto Complex with Pygeum, Saw Palmetto Standardized Extract (80 mg/softgel)	Mfd. for Puritans' Pride, Inc.
Quanterra Prostate Saw Palmetto Standardized Extract (160 mg/softgel)	Dist: Warner-Lambert Consumer Healthcare
Shaklee Formulas Saw Palmetto Plus, Saw Palmetto Standardized Extract (160 mg/softgel)	Dist: Shaklee Corp.

(continued)

Product name (concentration/pill)	Manufacturer (Mf) or distributor (Dist)
Spring Valley Saw Palmetto Extract (80 mg/softgel)	Mf: NaturPharma®
Sundown Herbals Standardized Saw Palmetto Extract (with berry) (225 mg/capsule)	Mf: Sundown Vitamins
Super Saw Palmetto (160 mg/softgel capsule)*	Mfd. for Enzymatic Therapy
Walgreens Saw Palmetto Standardized Extract (160 mg/softgel)	Dist: Walgreen Co.

* Tested through ConsumerLab.com's Ad Hoc Testing Program (Product was tested at the manufacturer's request after the initial review was completed and released.)

Copyright ConsumerLab.com, LLC, 2000, 2001. 2002, 2003. All rights reserved. Not to be reproduced, excerpted, or cited without written permission from ConsumerLab.com LLC.

CONSUMERTIPS™ FOR BUYING AND USING

ConsumerLab.com has prepared numerous important tips about dosing, selecting, and buying saw palmetto supplements. This information — along with our list of approved-quality brands — provides a valuable guide for choosing appropriate products.

Consumers seeking products most similar to those studied clinically should look for saw palmetto berry extract products, rather than crushed berry (nonextract) products. Look, too, for products containing fatty acids and sterols standardized for the specific compounds tested for in this review. In general, these will appear on labels as a minimum of 85% fatty acids and a minimum of 0.2% sterols. (See Expected fatty acids and sterols, page 149.) For example, a 160-mg pill of saw palmetto extract will have a minimum of 136 mg of fatty acids and 0.32 mg of sterols per pill.

The standard dosage of saw palmetto extract is 320 mg, usually taken as 160 mg twice per day. For crushed berry products (not extracts), the dosage is 1 to 2 grams of berry per day. Improvements may not be noticeable for at least 6 to 8 weeks and may take up to 3 to 4 months. Further improvements may be seen throughout the first 12 months.

CAUTIONS AND CONCERNS

Saw palmetto is generally safe when taken in appropriate amounts, but tell your physician if you're taking the herb and be aware that it can cause nausea and abdominal pain.

Furthermore, a proper diagnosis by a physician is important before using saw palmetto because the typical symptoms of enlarged prostate may signal other, more serious conditions that require prompt treatment. Saw palmetto isn't a treatment for prostate cancer.

Expected fatty acids* and sterols**

Individual fatty acids **	Formula	Percentage
Caproic Acid	$C_6H_{12}O_2$	0.3–0.8
Caprylic Acid	$C_8H_{16}O_2$	1.0–3.0
Capric Acid	$C_{10}H_{20}O_2$	1.0–3.0
Lauric Acid	$C_{12}H_{24}O_2$	25.0–32.0
Myristic Acid	$C_{14}H_{28}O_2$	10.0–15.0
Palmitic Acid	$C_{16}H_{32}O_2$	7.0–11.0
Stearic Acid	$C_{18}H_{36}O_2$	1.0–2.0
Oleic Acid	$C_{18}H_{34}O_2$	26.0–35.0
cis-Linoleic Acid	$C_{18}H_{32}O_2$	3.0–5.0
Linolenic Acid	$C_{18}H_{30}O_2$	0.5–1.5
Total:		**85.0% to 95.0%****
Individual Sterols: **		
Campesterol	$C_{28}H_{48}O$	0.01–0.1
Stigmasterol	$C_{29}H_{48}O$	0.01–0.1
Beta-sitosterol	$C_{29}H_{50}O$	0.1–0.4
Total:		**0.2% to 0.5%*****

* Based on extracts. For products containing berry powder only, total and individual constituents should be 10% of the extract values on a weight basis.
** Based on industry specification standards
*** United States Pharmacopoeia (proposed levels)

Soy & red clover isoflavones

WHAT IT IS

Isoflavones are phytoestrogens found in soy and red clover. Phytoestrogens are estrogen-like plant compounds that act like the hormone estrogen, although they are weaker than estrogen itself.

WHAT IT DOES

Much of the research on the health benefits of isoflavones is based on foods containing soy protein. Isoflavones are bound to soy protein; however, soy also contains other compounds that may have health benefits. For this reason, experts are uncertain whether the isoflavones themselves are responsible for the effects associated with soy.

Soy protein has been shown to reduce menopausal symptoms such as hot flashes, although not as much as estrogen replacement therapy. Intake of soy protein has also been found to help reduce total levels of cholesterol and LDLs (low-density lipoproteins, the "bad" cholesterol), while increasing levels of HDLs (high-density lipoproteins, the "good" cholesterol). In fact, the U.S. Food and Drug Administration (FDA) allows products that contain at least 6.25 grams of soy protein per serving and that are low in fat and cholesterol to declare that they can help reduce the risk of heart disease. This lipid-lowering effect hasn't been found with isoflavones alone, although soy proteins with higher levels of isoflavones have a greater lipid-lowering effect. Similarly, soy isoflavones, when used as supplements to foods containing soy protein, have been shown to maintain and even increase bone density. Soy isoflavones, which also act as antioxidants, may help prevent breast and prostate cancer. However, there is concern that large amounts of soy may not be safe for women with estrogen receptor-positive breast cancer or for pregnant or breast-feeding women.

Other plants, such as kudzu (Pueraria lobata) and red clover, also contain isoflavones. But clinical research specifically with kudzu has been limited, and it's technically difficult to measure some of its unique isoflavones. Studies indicate that red clover isoflavones may reduce menopausal symptoms, but results have varied. Red clover may also help maintain the bone density in the lower spine in perimenopausal and menopausal women, although not in postmenopausal women. Red clover isoflavones don't appear to reduce cholesterol levels, though both red clover and soy isoflavones may improve blood-vessel elasticity in perimenopausal and menopausal women. Ironically, isoflavones have an antiestrogen effect when the body's estrogen levels are high because isoflavones and estrogen compete for estrogen receptors. This may explain the lower incidence of breast cancer in populations with high intakes of soy foods and a possible beneficial effect of isoflavones in treating breast pain associated with the menstrual cycle.

A synthetic form of isoflavone, called ipriflavone—also available in supplement form—has the bone-stimulating effect of natural isoflavones but lacks other estrogen-like effects. However, a recent study found no significant reduction in bone loss in postmenopausal women taking ipriflavone. Moreover, ipriflavone might have been responsible for a reduction in white blood cells among study participants, a finding that concerned the researchers. Ipriflavone isn't intended for treating menopausal symptoms, and may not adversely affect estrogen receptor-positive breast cancer. Ipriflavone products weren't included in this review.

QUALITY CONCERNS

Because no government agency is responsible for routinely testing isoflavone supplements for their contents or quality, ConsumerLab.com independently evaluated several leading isoflavone products to determine whether they contained the type and quantity of isoflavones stated on their labels.

PRODUCT TESTING

ConsumerLab.com purchased 18 supplements containing soy isoflavones or red clover isoflavones. According to their labels, 12 products were made from soy isoflavones, 2 were made from red clover isoflavones, and 4 were made from combinations of soy and red clover isoflavones. The products were tested for their total isoflavone content (specifically glucosidic and aglycone forms of the isoflavones). (See "ConsumerLab.com's testing methods and standards," page 169.)

TEST FINDINGS

Of the 18 products tested, 5 didn't pass because they contained only 50% to 80% of the isoflavone amounts stated on the labels — 2 were combination products, 1 was a red clover product, and the remaining 2 were soy products.

Surprisingly, nearly all products claiming specific levels of aglycone isoflavones, such as genistein or daidzein, failed to meet their claims (and, consequently, didn't pass the review). However, among the passing products, aglycone isoflavones accounted for at least two-thirds of the total isoflavone amounts of stated on the labels.

QUALITY PRODUCTS

Listed alphabetically by name on pages 153 to 154 are the products that passed ConsumerLab.com's independent testing of soy and red clover isoflavone dietary supplements (see Soy & red clover isoflavones approved-quality products).

CONSUMERTIPS ™ FOR BUYING AND USING

ConsumerLab.com has prepared numerous important tips about dosing, selecting, and buying soy & red clover isoflavones supplements. This information — along with our list of approved-quality brands — provides a valuable guide for choosing appropriate products.

Manufacturers currently describe the isoflavone content of products in several ways: The term isoflavone can refer to either the aglycone form (meaning "without sugar") or to a larger compound that includes the isoflavone molecule and a sugar molecule, which together are referred to as a glycosidic isoflavone or isoflavone glycoside. Nearly all products contain a mixture of both forms. However, some products specifically declare the weight of the active aglycone isoflavone in the product,

Soy & red clover isoflavones approved-quality products

Product name (concentration of isoflavone/pill)	Manufacturer (Mf) or distributor (Dist)	Isoflavone sources
Soy Products		
GNC Natural Brand™ Soy Preventive Dietary Supplement (4.25 mg/capsule)	Dist: General Nutrition Corporation	Soy
Healthy Woman® Soy Menopause Supplement (55 mg/tablet)	Dist: Personal Products Company Division of McNeil-PPC, Inc.	Soy
Nature Made® Soy 50, 50 mg Soy Isoflavones Dietary Supplement (50 mg/tablet) ‡	Dist: Nature Made Nutritional Products	Soy
Nature's Resource® Soy Isoflavones (50 mg/capsule)* ‡	Dist: Nature's Resource	Soy
Nutrilite® Black Cohosh and Soy (16.6 mg/tablet) ‡	Mf: Nutrilite, Div. of Access Business Group International, LLC (formerly Amway)	Soy
Safeway Select™ Standardized Herbal Extract, Menopause Support, Soy Isoflavones 50 mg Concentrate Dietary Supplement (50 mg/caplet)	Dist: Safeway Inc.	Soy
Soy Care™ Dietary Supplement for Menopause (25 mg/capsule)	Mf: Inverness Medical, Inc.	Soy
Spring Valley Soy Isoflavones (40 mg/tablet)	Mf: NBTY	Soy
Sundown® Concentrated Soy Isoflavones (40 mg/capsule)	Mfd. for distribution by: Sundown Vitamins	Soy
VitaSmart® Soy Formula Dietary Supplement for Bone Health, Soy Isoflavones with Calcium and Vitamin D (45 mg/caplet)	Dist: Kmart Corporation	Soy
USANA® PhytoEstrin Dietary Supplement (14 mg/tablet)	USANA, Inc.	Soy

(continued)

Product name (concentration of isoflavone/pill)	Manufacturer (Mf) or distributor (Dist)	Isoflavone sources
Red Clover Products		
Promensil™, Non-GMO, A dietary supplement of plant estrogens extracted from red clover (40 mg/tablet)	Dist: Novogen, Inc.	Red Clover
Combination Products		
Shaklee® PhytoFem™ Black Cohosh, Soy Isoflavones, Flaxseed, & more Dietary Supplement (15 mg/capsule)	Dist: Shaklee Corp	Soy, Red Clover
Vitamin World® Red Clover Support Complex (40 mg/tablet)	Mf: Vitamin World, Inc.	Red Clover, Soy

* Tested through ConsumerLab.com's Ad Hoc Testing Program (Product was tested at the manufacturer's request after the initial review was completed and released.)
‡ See "More Brand Information," page 191.

though most include the weight of the attached sugar molecules, resulting in uncertainty over the actual amount of aglycone isoflavone present. Aglycone isoflavones may also be referred to by their specific names, which for soy are genistein, daidzein, and glycitein (note that all three end with the letters ein) and for red clover are biochanin A and formononetin. Similarly, the larger, sugar-containing, glycosidic isoflavones can be referred to by their specific names—that is, genistin, daidzin, and glycitin (all ending in in). Unfortunately, most products specifically stating levels of aglycone isoflavones didn't meet their claims.

Some products also claim to contain black cohosh, which may have a positive effect on menopause-related sleep disorders, mood disturbance, and hot flashes; however, studies have been limited, and its safety hasn't been evaluated beyond 6 months of use. Black cohosh shouldn't be confused with blue cohosh, which may be toxic.

The recommended daily dosage for treating menopausal symptoms is 50 mg of soy isoflavones or 40 mg of red clover isoflavones—both based on aglycone isoflavones. However, ConsumerLab's findings indicate that if a product claims to contain 50 mg of total isoflavones, for example, it may contain only about 40 mg of aglycone isoflavones—a factor that should be considered when figuring dosage.

Products themselves vary significantly in their suggested daily intake, ranging from as little as 8 mg to as much as 100 mg of isoflavones per day.

Desired effects — especially reducing hot flashes — may not be apparent for a few weeks.

Maintaining a relatively constant level of isoflavones in the body may be beneficial. If possible, divide the daily dose in two. In addition, taking isoflavones with a meal high in carbohydrates may aid absorption.

Currently, the average U.S. dietary intake of soy protein is low. But including more isoflavones in our diet may be a good thing. As stated by the FDA, "Consuming 25 grams of soy protein daily, as part of a diet low in saturated fat and cholesterol, may reduce the risk of heart disease." In countries where soy is a staple, such as Japan, 50 mg or more a day of isoflavones are routinely consumed. To obtain isoflavones directly from foods, consume foods and beverages made from soy protein. Be sure to look for soy protein isolate, which is rich in isoflavones. Because of processing differences, soy protein concentrate isn't as rich a source. (See Isoflavone content of selected foods, page 156.)

CAUTIONS AND CONCERNS

Isoflavones are generally safe when taken in appropriate amounts, but be aware that large doses should be avoided: animal research indicates that consuming excessive amounts could have adverse effects, such as reduced fertility.

Soy products and isoflavone supplements may be unsafe for women with estrogen receptor-positive breast cancer or for pregnant or breast-feeding women.

People who have impaired thyroid function should be aware that isoflavones can affect thyroid function.

People with allergies or hypersensitivity to soy products may have a similar reaction to foods or supplements containing isolated soy isoflavones.

Isoflavone content of selected foods

Here's a list of soy-based foods and estimates of their aglycone isoflavone content per 100 grams (about 3 $\frac{1}{2}$ oz). Be aware that soy oils and soy lecithin are devoid of isoflavones, and soy sauce contains only a very small amount.

Food:	Isoflavones (aglycone) per 100 grams
Soy flour (roasted)	199 mg
Soy flour (textured)	148 mg
Soy beans dry roasted	128 mg
Soy protein concentrate (aqueous washed)	102 mg
Soy protein isolate	97 mg
Soy beans cooked and boiled	55 mg
Tempeh	44 mg
Miso	43 mg
Tofu	31 mg
Soybean curd cheese	28 mg
Soy protein concentrate (produced by alcohol extraction)	12 mg
Soy milk (3.4 fl oz)	10 mg
Soy noodles	9 mg
Vegetable protein burger	8 mg

Source: USDA–Iowa State University Database on the Isoflavone Content of Foods, Release 1.2—2000.

St. John's wort

WHAT IT IS

As a dietary supplement, St. John's wort is widely used in the United States for treating mild to moderate depression as well as for relieving depression-related anxiety. The supplement hasn't been shown to be effective for treating severe depression.

WHAT IT DOES

Exactly how St. John's wort works is a mystery; what's more, researchers aren't certain which chemical component is most responsible for the antidepressant effects. However, most St. John's wort supplements come from concentrated extracts of the herb, and most clinical studies have used products standardized to contain hypericin or hyperforin. These compounds, therefore, can serve as markers for evaluating the quality of a St. John's wort product.

Although the flowers, leaves, and stem — collectively referred to as the aerial (aboveground) portion of St. John's wort — have all been used medicinally, the flowers have the highest concentration of hypericin.

QUALITY CONCERNS

During the growing season, St. John's wort accumulates cadmium, a carcinogen and kidney toxin, from the environment. Although the levels of cadmium in a supplement would be small and unlikely to cause disease, any quantity contributes to the daily intake. Besides, the safety margin between exposure in the normal diet and the levels that can produce deleterious effects is relatively small. Choosing a product with a low cadmium level is, therefore, best. Extracts, although concentrated, usually have the lowest cadmium levels because the extraction process removes some of the metal.

Because no government agency is responsible for routinely testing St. John' wort supplements for their contents or quality, ConsumerLab.com independently evaluated several leading St. John's wort products to determine whether they contained the St. John's wort amount stated on their labels.

PRODUCT TESTING

ConsumerLab.com purchased 21 brands of St. John's wort products; 18 claimed to contain standardized extracts, and 3 claimed to be combinations of extract and raw herb. All but 3 products made claims about hypericin content, and 2 products made claims for both hypericin and hyperforin content. All but 4 of the 21 products also identified the portion of the St. John's wort plant used, such as the flower, flower and leaves, or aerial portions. The products were tested for total hypericin, total hyperforin (if claimed) and contamination with the heavy metal, cadmium. (See "ConsumerLab.com's testing methods and standards," page 169.)

TEST FINDINGS

Of the 21 products tested, one-third, or 7, didn't pass because they didn't meet one or more of the following criteria: 4 products had levels of hypericin that ranged from 77% to 85% of their labeled amounts (or, if not labeled, of the minimum acceptable amount set by ConsumerLab.com for this review). These included 2 of the 3 products claiming a mixture of extract and raw herb, 1 of which claimed to contain hyperforin and actually contained only 21.7% of the labeled amount.

Five products contained levels of cadmium that exceeded acceptable levels, 3 of which had more than twice the acceptable amount. Although none of these 5 products alone would pose a serious health risk, they represent avoidable sources of cadmium. This group included all 3 extract/raw herb products, as well as 2 other products that had insufficient hypericin levels.

All 5 products claiming to be made from flowers passed. In addition,

4 out of 5 products labeled as made from flowers and leaves passed. Among the 7 products made from aerial portions — that is, any combination of flower, leaves, and stems — only 2 passed.

Ironically, all 3 products that didn't claim a specific hypericin or hyperforin level passed, whereas 5 of 18 products stating the levels failed. Products most likely to have passed testing claim to be made from St. John's wort flower or flower and leaves; products less likely to have passed, from aerial plant parts (a more general term that may include stems, for example) and were also more likely to contain raw herb as an ingredient.

QUALITY PRODUCTS
Listed alphabetically by name are the products that passed ConsumerLab.com's independent testing of St. John's wort dietary supplements (see St. John's wort approved-quality products, pages 160 to 161.)

CONSUMERTIPS™ FOR BUYING AND USING
ConsumerLab.com has prepared numerous important tips about dosing, selecting, and buying St. John's wort supplements. This information—along with our list of approved-quality brands—provides a valuable guide for choosing appropriate products.

Ideally, labels on St. John's wort products should indicate the amount of raw herb or extract per tablet in milligrams or grams. In addition, products should specify the concentration of total hypericin (0.3% by weight for extracts and 0.1% to 0.15% for raw herb, American Herbal Pharmacopoeia) or hyperforin (1% to 6% by weight for extracts). Label information, however, isn't a guarantee of quality.

Products claiming to contain St. John's wort flowers or flowers and leaves may be of higher quality than versions claiming to contain aerial plant parts (a more general term that may include stems). In addition, products made from the raw herb, instead of an extract, may have higher levels of cadmium.

St. John's wort preparations shown to be effective in clinical trials contained 0.2 to 1.0 mg of total hypericin per daily dose (German Commission E), 2 to 4 grams of the raw herb (dried, aboveground parts) per day, or 500 to 1,000 mg/day of standardized extract. However, a

St. John's wort approved-quality products

Product name (amount/pill)	Manufacturer (Mf) or distributor (Dist)
Enzymatic Therapy® St. John's Wort Extract With 4% Hyperforin, Standardized Potency (300 mg extract/capsule)	Mf: Enzymatic Therapy
Harmonex™ for emotional and physical harmony St. John's Wort with Siberian Ginseng Standardized Herbal Supplement (450 mg extract/caplet)	Dist: Chattem, Inc.
HealthSmart Vitamins® St. John's Wort (450 mg extract/capsule)	Dist: HealthSmart Vitamins
Herbalife® Advanced St. John's Wort with Uplifting Herbs Dietary Supplement (300 mg extract/tablet)	Dist: Herbalife International of America, Inc.
Herb Tech™ *Hypericum perforatum* St. John's Wort 300 mg, Standardized Extract, Standardized to contain 0.3% Hypericin (300 mg extract/capsule)	Mf: Vitamin World, Inc.
Kira® St. John's Wort Dietary Supplement Exclusive LI 160™ Formula (300 mg extract/tablet)	Dist: Lichtwer Pharma U.S., Inc.
Longs® St. John's Wort 300 mg Standardized Extract Herbal Supplement (300 mg extract/capsule)	Dist: Longs Drug Stores
Movana™ Advanced St. John's Wort Mood Support Dietary Supplement (300 mg extract/tablet)	Dist: Pharmaton Natural Health Products
Nature Made® Herbs St. John's Wort 300 mg Supplement Standardized Extract (300 mg extract/tablet)* ‡	Dist: Nature Made
Nature's Bounty® Herbal Harvest® St. John's Wort 300mg, Standardized to contain 0.3% Hypericin (300 mg extract/capsule)	Mf: Nature's Bounty, Inc.
Nature's Plus® Herbal Actives St. John's Wort 300mg Standardized Botanical Supplement, 0.3–0.5% Hypericin (300 mg extract/capsule)	Mf: Nature's Plus

(continued)

St John's wort

Product name (amount/pill)	Manufacturer (Mf) or distributor (Dist)
Nature's Resource Herbal Supplement St. John's Wort 300 mg Extract (300 mg extract/capsule)* ‡	Dist: Nature's Resource
Nutrilite® St. John's Wort with Lemon Balm (300 mg extract/capsule) ‡	Mf: Nutrilite, a Division of Access Business Group International LLC
One A Day® Tension and Mood with St. John's Wort and Natural Kava Kava (225 mg extract/tablet)	Dist: Bayer Corporation
Sundown Herbals Standardized St. John's Wort, Standardized Extract Containing Hypericin Plus Flavonoids and Proanthocyanidins Herbal Supplement (150 mg extract/capsule)	Dist: Sundown Vitamins
Yerba Prima® St. John's Wort Extra Strength Herbal Supplement (450 mg extract/capsule)	Dist: Yerba Prima

* Tested through ConsumerLab.com's Ad Hoc Testing Program (Proudct was tested at the manufacturer's request after the initial review was completed and released.)
‡ See "More Brand Information," page 191.

dosage of 900 mg/day of extract, standardized to 0.3% hypericin, is most commonly recommended, usually in 300-mg doses three times a day.

Among the products evaluated, the doses of extract recommended by the manufacturers varied from as little as 175 mg/day to the more common 900 mg/day. Consequently, when selecting a product, compare the costs for equivalent daily doses, such as 900 mg/day, rather than the number of recommended daily servings per container.

Desired effects may take up to 4 weeks to become apparent.

CAUTIONS AND CONCERNS
St. John's wort is generally safe when taken in appropriate amounts, but be aware it can interact with other drugs, such as monoamine oxidase inhibitors and selective serotonin reuptake inhibitors. It may reduce the

effectiveness of drugs such as protease inhibitors, cyclosporine, digoxin, warfarin (Coumadin), chemotherapy, contraceptives, antipsychotics, cholesterol-lowering drugs, and theophylline, and it may interfere with the absorption of iron and other minerals. St. John's wort shouldn't be taken with antimigraine drugs or other antidepressants.

In rare cases, St. John's wort may cause abdominal discomfort and, in doses exceeding the normal 900 mg/day, sensitivity to sunlight. This sensitivity may increase if the supplement is taken with other drugs causing sensitivity to light.

Because of all these actions and interactions, individuals should discuss using St. John's wort with their physician before taking it.

The safety of St. John's wort hasn't been well evaluated in children or during pregnancy or breast-feeding. Therefore, it isn't recommended for women who may become pregnant.

Valerian

WHAT IT IS

A popular herb, valerian is used as a calmative and a sleep-promoting sedative. Valerian dietary supplements should be made from the root (or rhizomes) of Valeriana officinalis.

WHAT IT DOES

Valerian appears to target the central nervous system neurotransmitter gamma-aminobutyric acid as do most prescription tranquilizers.

QUALITY CONCERNS

Like other herbal ingredients, valerian root has many chemical components. Although it isn't clear which chemicals are key to its effectiveness, certain "valerenic acids" have been associated with quality valerian and are, therefore, considered to be excellent marker compounds for testing valerian products. Most clinical research has been conducted with V. officinalis. Products made from other species can be rich in didrovaltrate, which may be toxic to cells, according to laboratory testing.

Because no government agency is responsible for routinely testing valerian supplements for their contents or quality, ConsumerLab.com independently evaluated several leading valerian products for valerenic acid to determine whether they contained the valerian type and amount stated on their labels.

PRODUCT TESTING

ConsumerLab.com purchased 17 valerian products: 7 valerian extracts,

6 valerian powders, and 4 combinations of the 2. Although most products stated that they contained only valerian, 5 listed one or more additional herbs, such as kava kava, hops, lemon balm, and skullcap. All had adequate labeling indicating the proper species and plant part as well as the valerian amount, and 8 also claimed to be standardized to provide specific levels of valerenic acids. The products were tested for their valerenic acid content. (See "ConsumerLab.com's testing methods and standards," page 169.)

TEST FINDINGS

Of the 17 products tested, only 9 passed. Of the 8 that failed, 4 had no detectable levels of the valerenic acids and another 4 had about half the stated amounts. The 6 products that were made exclusively from root powder had the worst results: only 1 passed. Of the 7 products made from extract alone, 4 passed. All 4 of the combined powder and extract products passed the tests.

ConsumerLab.com used a European standard for calculating valerenic acid levels that's somewhat more stringent than that generally used in the United States. However, all the failing products would have failed using either standard. Why so many products lacked the claimed valerian is a mystery. Perhaps the wrong species had been used — and, perhaps, good manufacturing practices (testing ingredients before processing) could have prevented the problem.

QUALITY PRODUCTS

Listed alphabetically by name on page 166 are the products that passed ConsumerLab.com's independent testing of valerian dietary supplements (see Valerian approved-quality products).

CONSUMERTIPS™

ConsumerLab.com has prepared numerous important tips about dosing, selecting, and buying valerian supplements. This information — along with our list of approved-quality brands — provides a valuable guide for choosing appropriate products.

Consumers should expect valerian product labels to specify the species of valerian (V. officinalis, although the claim of "valerian" also denotes this species), part of the plant used (root or rhizomes), form (powder, extract, or tincture), and dose in grams or milligrams.

The concentration of total valerenic acids should also be indicated—ideally, at least 0.17% for root powders or proportionately higher for extracts, which are typically 0.8% valerenic acids. These are calculated on a weight basis.

Appropriate dosages depend on the form and concentration of valerian in the supplement: to treat insomnia, the standard daily dose of valerian root powder is 2 to 3 grams, although it's proportionately less for extracts. For example, the daily dose for an extract standardized to 0.8% valerenic acids would be 400 to 600 mg. The dose should be taken 30 to 60 minutes before bedtime. To treat anxiety, up to twice the daily dose used for insomnia is recommended, but this dose should be taken in two to three divided doses during the day. Some experts suggest taking lower doses of valerian when also using products containing other ingredients believed to have tranquilizing effects, such as hops. Consequently, the appropriate daily dose of valerian may vary considerably. Among the products evaluated, for example, dosages recommended by the manufacturers ranged from 200 to 1,000 mg/day among extracts to from 1,000 mg (1 g) to 8,000 mg (8 g)/day for powder-based products.

Although some clinical trials report fast-onset of action, full effects of valerian may take 2 to 4 weeks.

Valerian extracts and powders typically have a musty odor, and it's common for products to have flavors added, such as spearmint, peppermint, and vanilla, to help mask the odor. Many valerian products also claim to contain other herbs with potential sedative effects, such as kava kava, lemon balm, and hops.

CAUTIONS AND CONCERNS
Valerian products from the species V. officinalis are believed to be safe at recommended doses, but be aware that valerian can cause minor gastrointestinal upset. It can also, in rare cases, have a mild stimulant effect. Long-term use may occasionally cause headache, restlessness, and

Valerian approved-quality products

Product name, (form and amount/pill)[1]	Manufacturer (Mf) or distributor (Dist)
Celestial Seasoning® Sleepytime Extra™ Ultimate Blend with Valerian (root extract and powder; 187.5 mg/capsule)	Mf: Celestial Seasonings, Inc.
Eckerd® Standardized Herbal Extract Valerian 100 mg (root extract; 100 mg/caplet)	Dist: Eckerd Drug Comp.
Nature's Resource® Herbal Supplement Valerian (root extract 100 mg/softgel)* ‡	Dist: Nature's Resource Products
Nature's Resource® Premium Herb Standardized Valerian (root powder; 530 mg/capsule)*	Dist: Nature's Resource Products
Nutrilite Valerian and Hops (150 mg root extract and 50 mg root powder/tablet) ‡	Dist: Access Business Group International LLC
Planetary Formulas® Valerian Easy Sleep™ (26.5 mg root extract and 132.5 mg root powder/tablet)	Dist: Planetary Formulas
Pharmanex® Valerian (root extract; 350 mg/capsule)	Dist: Pharmanex
Ricola® Herbal Health™ Night Time Formula with Valerian—Kava Kava (root extract; 200 mg/tablet)	Dist: Ricola, Inc.
Sedonium Valerian Extract, Exclusive LI 156 Formula (root extract; 300 mg/tablet)	Dist: Lichtwer Pharma U.S., Inc.
Swanson Ultra™ Standardized Valerian (200 mg root extract and 300 mg root powder/capsule)	Dist: Swanson Health Products

* Tested through ConsumerLab.com's Ad Hoc Testing Program (Product was tested at the manufacturer's request after the initial review was completed and released.)

‡ See "More Brand Information," page 191.

[1]Unless otherwise indicated, extracts in all products were 0.8% valerenic acids on a % wt/wt basis (which may also be stated as a 6:1 extract).

dilation of the pupils. Although valerian may impair attention when used during wakeful hours, it doesn't seem to cause drowsiness upon waking after use for insomnia.

Valerian affects the central nervous system and may have an additive effect when used with other tranquilizers, such as benzodiazepines and barbiturates. It, therefore, shouldn't be taken with these drugs. Valerian shouldn't be used with alcohol.

Skullcap is sometimes used in valerian products. However, its effectiveness isn't well proven, and some valerian-skullcap combination products have resulted in liver toxicity, according to reports. Possibly, substitution of the liver-toxic herb germander for the skullcap caused the problem. (See "Herbal alert," pages 21 to 26.)

The safety of valerian hasn't been well evaluated for children or for women who are pregnant or breast-feeding. Therefore, valerian isn't recommended for use by such individuals or by women who may become pregnant.

APPENDICES

ConsumerLab.com's testing methods and standards

For each review, ConsumerLab.com evaluated the products using the best testing methods and standards available at the time. Consequently, many of the tests used surpassed the requirements of the U.S. Food and Drug Administration (FDA). All products were tested to determine whether they contained the main ingredient specified on the label. On supplements prone to having specific problems, additional tests were performed. Details of testing for each product review are given below.

Products passing ConsumerLab.com's evaluations had to meet specific criteria in either a first or second round of testing. Passing scores in each analysis included margins of technical error. In addition, ConsumerLab.com reserved the right to disqualify a product at any time if the product seemed to be unsafe or to provide misleading or inaccurate label information. Testing evolved over a three-year period, so methods and standards vary, depending on the time of the test.

Multivitamins & multiminerals

ConsumerLab.com purchased 27 brands of multivitamin and multimineral products: 15 general multis (no specified age or gender category, but evaluated only for adult use), 2 prenatal multis, 3 women's multis, 2 senior's multis (generally for people ages 50 and older), and

5 children's multis. These products were tested for their amounts of several common labeled ingredients: folic acid, calcium, and vitamin A (retinol and beta-carotene). Because not all products were labeled to contain every one of these ingredients, some products were alternatively tested for other ingredients — for example, vitamin C (ascorbic acid) if folic acid wasn't an ingredient, and iron or zinc if calcium wasn't an ingredient. Products were also tested for disintegration (excluding chewable and time-release products), lead contamination, and compliance with the most recent Dietary Reference Intakes (DRIs). The specific tests used to evaluate these products and the standards for passing the tests appear under "Testing methods" and "Passing score."

TESTING METHODS
Each product was tested for at least one index element in each category. The first element within each category was selected unless it wasn't claimed to be in the product, in which case, the next claimed element was selected.

Oil-soluble vitamins
Vitamin A (beta carotene and
   retinol [retinyl acetate or
   palmitate] evaluated
   independently)
Vitamin E (natural and
   synthetic forms)
Vitamin D

Water-soluble vitamins
Folic acid (folate)
Vitamin C (ascorbic acid)

B Vitamins
Niacin
Pyridoxine
Riboflavin

Minerals
Calcium
Iron
Zinc
Magnesium

Products were analyzed for their vitamin and mineral index elements using the USP (United States Pharmacopeia) 24th edition, Methods for Oil- and Water-Soluble Vitamins and Mineral Tablets in an independent laboratory.

Disintegration of nonchewable and non–time-release products was analyzed using USP <2040> recommendations entitled "Disintegration and Dissolution of Nutritional Supplements."

Analyses for lead were performed using an atomic absorption or graphite furnace method or ICP-MS (inductively coupled plasma-mass spectroscopy).

Products failing either the content or disintegration test were sent to another independent laboratory for a second round of testing. Independent laboratories conducted all tests without knowing the identities of the products.

PASSING SCORE

To receive a passing score, a product had to meet these criteria in either a first or second round of testing:

• contain at least 100% but no more than 150% of its claimed amount of the index elements. Any product claiming to have vitamin A had to meet its claimed amount for total vitamin A (beta-carotene and retinol combined) as well as meet any claimed ratio of beta-carotene to total vitamin A.

• meet recommended USP parameters for disintegration for vitamin supplements (excluding chewable and time-release products) and contain less than 3 mcg of lead per serving per day. (Reference: The FDA hasn't established lead limits for dietary supplements, but ConsumerLab.com's limit is roughly equivalent to those established by the USP and the International Food Chemicals Codex: 3 parts/million for lead in calcium carbonate supplements. The state of California has established a limit of 0.5 mcg of lead per day for any multivitamin, although this limit is raised when certain minerals are in the product.)

• clearly and accurately state the amount of vitamins and minerals (oil- and water-soluble) in the product..

Products were retested in a second independent laboratory. For a product to fail, it had to have a failing result in at least one criteria in the second evaluation. A product that passed the above criteria but exceeded the Upper Tolerable Intake Level (UL), established by the Institute of Medicine of the National Academies, for any ingredient for the product's intended population was classified as conditionally approved and received an explanatory footnote.

Passing scores allow for specific margins of technical error associated with each analysis.

B vitamins (thiamin, riboflavin, niacin, pantothenic acid, B_6, folic acid, B_{12}, and biotin)

ConsumerLab.com purchased 21 dietary supplements claiming to contain single B vitamins or B-vitamin complexes and tested them for their levels of 7 of the 8 B vitamins: thiamin, riboflavin, total B_3 (niacin and niacinamide), total B_5 (pantothenic acid), total B_6 (pyridoxine and derivatives), folic acid, and total B_{12}. Their ability to break down in solution was evaluated as well. (Chewable and time-release products weren't tested for disintegration.) Biotin wasn't evaluated because no suitable analytical standard exists. The specific tests used to evaluate these products and the standards for passing the tests appear here under "Testing methods" and "Passing score."

TESTING METHODS

Product elements were analyzed using the United States Pharmacopeia (USP) <2040> Methods for Oil- and Water-Soluble Vitamins and Mineral Tablets in independent laboratories. Disintegration of nonchewable and nontime-release products was analyzed using USP recommendations entitled "Disintegration and Dissolution of Nutritional Supplements."

Independent laboratories conducted all tests without knowing the identities of the products.

PASSING SCORE

To receive a passing score, a product had to meet these criteria in either a first or second round of testing:
• contain at least 100% but no more than 150% of the B vitamins claimed
• meet recommended USP parameters for disintegration for vitamin supplements
• clearly and accurately state the amount of minerals and vitamins (oil and water soluble) in the product.

Retesting was performed in a second independent laboratory. A product that passed the above criteria but exceeded the UL for any ingredient for the product's intended population received an explanatory footnote.

Vitamin C

ConsumerLab.com purchased 26 brands of vitamin C products, including 5 products for children. Of these, 7 claimed USP quality on their labels. All were tested for their levels of vitamin C and their ability to break down in solution. Chewable and time-release products weren't tested for disintegration. The specific tests used to evaluate these products and the standards for passing the tests appear here under "Testing methods" and "Passing score."

TESTING METHODS

All products were analyzed using the AOAC (Association of Official Analytical Chemists) Official Method 43.064 — Microfluorometric Method for Quantitation of Vitamin C (ascorbic acid). Products not passing this initial assay were tested using an HPLC (high-performance liquid chromatography) assay. Disintegration of nonchewable and nontime-release products was analyzed using USP 2040 recommendations entitled "Disintegration and Dissolution of Nutritional Supplements." Products had two opportunities to pass the disintegration-and-dissolution test.

Any product that failed either the content or disintegration test was sent to another independent laboratory for the second round of testing. Independent laboratories conducted all tests without knowing the identities of the products.

PASSING SCORE

To receive a passing score, a product had to meet these criteria in either a first or second round of testing:
• clearly and accurately state the vitamin C amount in the product
• contain at least 100% but no more than 120% of its labeled vitamin C (allowing for a margin of error of 8% and 4% for the microfluorometric and HPLC methods, respectively)
• meet recommended USP parameters for disintegration for vitamin supplements (excluding chewable and time-release products).

Vitamin E

ConsumerLab.com purchased 28 different vitamin E products: 19 labeled as natural vitamin E, 8 capsules labeled as synthetic vitamin E, and 1 cream labeled as synthetic vitamin E. The products were tested to determine whether they correctly identified the vitamin E type and amount. The specific tests used to evaluate these products and the standards for passing the tests appear here under "Testing methods" and "Passing score."

TESTING METHODS

All products were first analyzed for various vitamin E forms including mixed tocopherols using a high-performance liquid chromatography (HPLC) assay in an independent laboratory.

Products not passing the initial assay were tested in a second independent laboratory, using a similar HPLC assay, the United States Pharmacopeia (USP) 24 assay.

In addition, products claiming to contain natural forms of vitamin E were analyzed by optical rotation, also using the USP 24 assay and a HPLC chiral separation.

Independent laboratories conducted all tests without knowing the identities of the products.

PASSING SCORE

To receive a passing score, a product had to meet these criteria in either a first or second round of testing:

• contain at least 100%, but no more than 120% of the claimed amount of vitamin E (allowing for a margin of error of 5% for the HPLC method)

• meet recommended USP parameters, if labeled as natural vitamin E, for the specific rotation for natural vitamin E supplements (not less than +24 degree [degree angle of rotation]) and contain no synthetic vitamin E. (Note that d-alpha-tocopheryl acid succinate and acetate are stabilized forms of natural vitamin E.)

• clearly and accurately state the amount of vitamin E in the product.
    Products were retested in a second independent laboratory.

Calcium

ConsumerLab.com purchased 35 brands of calcium-containing products, several of which also contained other vitamins or minerals, such as magnesium and vitamin D. The brands included 22 nonchewable calcium tablets, softgels, or syrups; 4 chewable antacid tablets; 2 adult chewable tablets or soft chews; 5 children's chewable tablets; and 2 calcium-fortified orange juices. Products were tested for calcium as well as contamination with lead, arsenic, cadmium, and aluminum. The specific tests used to evaluate these products and the standards for passing the tests appear here under "Testing methods" and "Passing score."

TESTING METHODS

Analyses for calcium and metals were first performed using an atomic absorption and graphite furnace method in an independent laboratory. Products not having enough calcium were retested in a second independent laboratory using the same method. Products found to be contaminated with metals were retested using ICP-MS (inductively coupled plasma-mass spectroscopy) in a third independent laboratory.

Independent laboratories conducted all tests without knowing the identities of the products.

PASSING SCORE

To receive a passing score, a product had to meet these criteria in either a first or second round of testing:
- contain at least 100% but no more than 150% of its labeled amount of elemental calcium
- meet purity standards for contamination by metals, including a lead level of less than 3 parts/million (7.5 mcg/gram of calcium) using the United States Pharmacopeia (USP) and the Food Chemicals Codex.
- meet purity standards for contamination by metals, including a cadmium level of less than 0.2 parts per million (micrograms per gram) using World Health Organization proposed guidelines for fruits, nuts, and vegetables; standards for dietary supplements are not available
- meet purity standards for contamination by metals, including arsenic levels of less than 10 mg/day/serving, using California guidelines.

Passing scores allowed for specific margins of technical error associated with each analysis.

Iron

ConsumerLab.com purchased 19 iron supplements, several of which included other nutrients, such as vitamin C, folic acid and other B vitamins, herbs, and calcium. These products were tested for their amount of iron, disintegration, and contamination with lead. The specific tests used to evaluate these products and the standards for passing the tests appear under "Testing methods" and "Passing score."

TESTING METHODS
Analyses for iron and lead were first performed using an atomic absorption and flame method and inductively coupled plasma-mass spectroscopy in an independent laboratory.

Products not having passing levels of iron as well as those contaminated with lead were retested for the specific metal using an atomic absorption/flame and atomic absorption/graphite furnace methods respectively in a second independent laboratory.

Disintegration of nonchewable and nontime release formulations was analyzed using USP (United States Pharmacopeia) <2040> recommendations entitled "Disintegration and Dissolution of Nutritional Supplements." Products failing to disintegrate properly were retested using the same method in a separate laboratory.

Independent laboratories conducted all tests without knowing the identities of the products.

PASSING SCORE
To receive a passing score, a product had to meet these criteria in either a first or second round of testing:
• contain at least 100% but no more than 125% of its labeled amount of elemental iron
• meet recommended USP parameters for disintegration of nutritional supplements (excluding chewable and time-release products)
• clearly and accurately state the amount of iron and other ingredients in the product, as required by the FDA

- contain less than 0.5 mcg of lead per the greater of either (a) 18 mg of elemental iron or (b) the product's maximum suggested daily serving (Note: California's Proposition 65 law requires products exceeding 0.5 mg of lead per suggested daily serving to carry a warning label.)
- provide proper packaging, such as child-resistant caps or blister packaging, for products containing 30 mg or more of iron per pill, to avoid accidental poisoning in children.

Passing scores allowed for specific margins of technical error associated with each analysis.

If the product contained herbs, it also needed to include the proper plant name, the plant part used (root/rhizome), the herb used form (root powder, extract, or tincture), and the amount of herb per pill or dose in grams or milligrams (1 gram = 1,000 mg).

Coenzyme Q10

ConsumerLab.com purchased 29 different CoQ10 products, several of which also contained other ingredients, such as bioflavonoids and vitamin E. The group contained these products: 17 softgels, 11 tablets or capsules, and 1 sublingual tablet. These products were tested for their claimed amount of CoQ10. The specific tests used to evaluate these products and the standards for passing the tests appear here under "Testing methods" and "Passing score."

TESTING METHODS

Analysis for CoQ10 was performed using an HPLC method (USP method for finished products) in an independent laboratory. Products with inappropriate levels of CoQ10 were then retested in a second independent laboratory using a comparable HPLC method.

Independent laboratories conducted all tests without knowing the identities of the products.

PASSING SCORE

To receive a passing score, a product had to meet these criteria in either a first of second round of testing:
- contain a minimum of 100% but no more than 150% of its labeled amount of CoQ10.

Retesting was performed in a second independent laboratory.

Creatine

ConsumerLab.com purchased 13 brands of creatine monohydrate supplements. The products were tested for creatine monohydrate and contamination with creatinine and dicyandiamide. The specific tests used to evaluate these products and the standards for passing the tests appear here under "Testing methods" and "Passing score."

TESTING METHODS

Analyses for creatine monohydrate was initially performed by capillary electrophoresis (CE). All products were also subjected to high-performance liquid chromatography (HPLC) to analyze again for creatine as well as for creatinine and dicyandiamide.

Any product not passing the first evaluation was sent to another independent laboratory to repeat HPLC testing for the criteria on which it didn't pass. The CE and HPLC methods are widely used in the industry and were internally verified. Independent laboratories conducted all tests without knowing the identities of the products.

PASSING SCORE

To receive a passing score, a product had to meet these criteria in either a first or second round of testing:
- meet its label claims for creatine monohydrate content and purity
- contain no less than 99.9% of the claimed amount of creatine monohydrate
- contain a combined weight of creatinine and dicyandiamide representing no more than 0.1% of the measured weight of the creatine monohydrate.

Echinacea

ConsumerLab.com purchased 25 echinacea products and tested them for 100% of the claimed amounts and types of echinacea, as well as the claimed levels of phenols (specifically caftaric acid, chlorogenic acid, echinacoside, and cichoric acid). If the phenol levels weren't clearly labeled, products were held to specific minimum standards consistent with clinical research on echinacea. Products were also required to meet purity requirements for microbial contamination. The specific tests used to evaluate these products and the standards for passing the tests appear here under "Testing methods" and "Passing score."

TESTING METHODS

All products were first analyzed for the phenolic constituents using a HPLC (high-performance liquid chromatography) assay in an independent laboratory.

Products not passing the initial assay were tested in a second independent laboratory using an HPLC assay developed by the Institute for Nutraceutical Advancement's Method Validation Program to specifically test for the presence and amount of caftaric acid, chlorogenic acid, echinacoside, and cichoric acid.

Analyses for microbial contaminants were made using methods from the FDA's Bacteriological Analytical Manual and included testing for Escherichia coli, Salmonella spp., Staphylococcus aureus, Pseudomonas aeruginosa, and other enteric bacteria, including Klebsiella, Enterobacter, Proteus, Citrobacter, Aerobacter, Providencia, and Serratia. Testing also included analyses for total aerobic bacteria, yeast, and mold.

Any product that didn't pass the microbial testing was sent to another independent laboratory for retesting. Independent laboratories conducted all tests without knowing the identities of the products.

PASSING SCORE

To receive a passing score, a product had to meet these criteria in either a first or second round of testing:
• clearly and accurately provide the label information required by the FDA—
  Species of echinacea used (E. purpurea, E. angustifolia, or E. pallida)
  Part of the plant used (root or aerial portions, which include the stem, leaves, and flowers and is also referred to as the "herb")
  Form of echinacea used (whole herb or root, extract, or tincture)
  Amount of echinacea per pill or dose in grams or milligrams (1 gram = 1,000 mg)
• meet its label claims for total phenolic content, with a minimum of 1% total phenols based on whole herb or root (The percentage is proportionally higher for extracts or tinctures, depending on their

level of concentration. Total phenols were calculated as the sum of caftaric acid, chlorogenic acid, echinacoside, and cichoric acid.)

- contain detectable levels of specific markers—

  Products labeled as containing the roots of E. angustifolia or E. pallida had to contain detectable levels of echinacoside.

  Products labeled as containing roots or herb of E. purpurea had contain detectable levels of cichoric, caftaric, and chlorogenic acids; however, if they were E. purpurea–only products, they could contain no more than trace levels of echinacoside.

- test negative for Escherichia coli, Salmonella spp., Staphylococcus aureus, and Pseudomonas aeruginosa (as required by the FDA). In addition, a product had to contain less than the following levels of microbes (as specified by the WHO, Quality Control Methods for Medicinal Plant Material, 1998)—

  100,000 microbes/gram of aerobic bacteria

  1,000 microbes/gram of yeast and mold

  1,000 microbes/gram of other coliform bacteria

  Passing scores allow for specific margins of technical error associated with each analysis.

Fish oils: Omega-3 fatty acids (EPA & DHA)

ConsumerLab.com purchased 20 omega-3 marine oil products, 19 of which were EPA/DHA combination products made from fish oils and one of which was a DHA-only product made from algal oil. These were tested for amounts of EPA and DHA, peroxide levels (which indicate spoilage), and contamination with mercury. The specific tests used to evaluate these products and the standards for passing the tests appear here under "Testing methods" and "Passing score."

TESTING METHODS

All products were analyzed for their EPA and DHA components by gas chromatography, using a modified Official Method 991.39 from the Association of Official Analytical Chemists, International.

Products not passing this initial assay for EPA and DHA were retested using modified AOCS (American Oil Chemists Society) methods for fatty acid determination. Peroxide values were analyzed using AOCS Methods CD 8-53 and 12-57. Products were tested for total mercury using a cold vapor atomic absorption method.

Any products that failed the initial analyses were retested on at least one criteria on which it didn't initially pass. Retesting was performed in a second independent laboratory. Independent laboratories conducted all tests without knowing the identities of the products.

PASSING SCORE

To receive a passing score, a product had to meet these criteria in either a first or second round of testing:
- contain 100% but no more than 150% of label claims for EPA and DHA
- meet standards for a peroxide value of no more than 10 meq/kg
- meet standards for total mercury content of less than 100 parts per billion (ppb).

Ginkgo biloba

ConsumerLab.com purchased 30 leading brands of ginkgo biloba and tested them for their amounts of flavonol glycosides and terpene lactones. The specific tests used to evaluate these products and the standards for passing the tests appear here under "Testing methods" and "Passing score."

TESTING METHODS

All products were analyzed using the Quantitative Analysis of Bilobalide and Ginkgolides (Terpene Lactones) by high-performance liquid chromatography (HPLC), using INA (Institute for Nutraceutical Advancement) or a comparable analytical method and the Quantitative Analysis of Flavonol Glycosides by HPLC as described in the INA, method.

Independent laboratories conducted all tests without knowing the identities of the products.

PASSING SCORE

To receive a passing score, a product had to meet these criteria:
- meet or exceed its label claims for ginkgo biloba

- suggest a daily dosage that would provide a clinically appropriate amount of GBE (the extract)
- meet or exceed the percentage of weight for flavonol glycosides and terpene lactones in GBE as shown†:

Ginkgo Flavonol Glycosides
    Quercetin   minimum 9.5% (wt/wt)
    Kaempferol   minimum 10.5% (wt/wt)
    Isorhamnetin   minimum 2% (wt/wt)

Terpene Lactones
    Ginkgolides A, B, C   minimum 2.8% (wt/wt)†
    Bilobalide   minimum 2.6% (wt/wt)†

†Source: German Commission E Monographs

Ginseng

ConsumerLab.com purchased 22 brands of Asian and American ginseng products and tested them for total ginsenosides and contamination with heavy metals and pesticides. The specific tests used to evaluate these products and the standards for passing the tests appear here under "Testing methods" and "Passing score."

TESTING METHODS

Analysis for ginsenosides was done by high-performance liquid chromatography, using the Ginseng Evaluation Program methods established by the American Botanical Council. This analysis specifically tests for the presence and amounts of the seven major types of ginsenosides. Based on the scientific literature, the weight of these ginsenosides is assumed to represent about 90% of the total ginsenosides in a product and is, therefore, used to calculate the total ginsenoside weight in products.

Analyses for the heavy metals arsenic, cadmium, and lead were performed using atomic absorption with a graphite furnace and inductively coupled plasma/mass spectroscopy.

Analyses for the pesticides quintozene (pentachloronitrobenzene), lindane (hexachlorocyclohexane), hexachlorobenzene, and related compounds (pentachloroaniline, pentachlorothioanisol, alpha-benzenehexachloride, beta-benzenehexachloride, delta-benzenehexachloride, and tetrachloroanaline) was performed using a modified method by gas chromatography with an electron capture detector or gas chromatography with mass spectroscopy/mass spectroscopy detection described in the U.S. Food and Drug Administration (FDA) Pesticide Analytical Manual and a modification of that method (presented at the Sept. 1999 AOAC, Houston, Tex., entitled "Trace Contaminants in Dietary Supplements: Pesticide Analysis in Ginseng").

Retesting for products that failed was performed in a second independent laboratory. Independent laboratories conducted all tests without knowing the identities of the products.

PASSING SCORE
To receive a passing score, a product had to meet these criteria in either a first or second round of testing:
• meet its label claims for ginsenoside content and, at a minimum, contain the following total ginsenosides, respective of the type of ginseng labeled: 1.5% Asian root powder (German Commission E recommendation), 3% Asian root extract (USP recommendation), 2% for American root powder, and 4% American root extract (common industry standard).
• contain less than 3 mcg of lead per serving per day (Reference: Although the FDA has not established lead limits for dietary supplements, ConsumerLab.com's limit is roughly equivalent to those established by the USP and the International Food Chemicals Codex, which have established limits of 3 parts per million for lead in calcium carbonate supplements. California has established strict standards for lead, including 0.5 mcg/serving/day for foods and 1.5 mcg/day for calcium supplements. Products sold in California that exceed these levels are required to carry warning labels.)
• contain less than 0.2 parts/million (or micrograms per gram) of cadmium (per World Health Organization proposed guidelines for fruits, nuts, and vegetables — standards for dietary supplements are not available)
• contain less than 10 mcg of arsenic per daily serving (California)
• contain less than 0.1 part/million of hexachlorobenzene,

1 part/million of quintozene (total of pentachloronitrobenzene [PCNB], pentachloroaniline and pentachlorothioanisol), and less than 0.6 part/million of lindane (USP/European Pharmacopeia)
• clearly and accurately state the amount of ginseng in the product.

Glucosamine & chondroitin

ConsumerLab.com purchased 25 brands of glucosamine, chondroitin, and combined glucosamine-chondroitin products and tested them for quality. The specific tests used to evaluate these products and the standards for passing the tests appear here under "Testing methods" and "Passing score."

TESTING METHODS
The best method for analyzing these products is under scientific debate. In our analyses, supplements containing glucosamine or chondroitin were first analyzed by capillary electrophoresis in an independent laboratory.

Products that didn't pass the initial test were reanalyzed using a colorimetric titration method in a second independent laboratory and, in the case of several products that contained chondroitin, were also retested using gel permeation chromatography (a type of high-performance liquid chromatography) in a third independent laboratory.

Independent laboratories conducted all tests without knowing the identities of the products.

PASSING SCORE
To receive a passing score, a product had to meet these criteria in either a first, second, or third round of testing:
• meet or exceed the claims on its label for the appropriate form of glucosamine, chondroitin, or both within a 5% margin of error after factoring in the contributed weight of salts or other listed ingredients (A product could pass with any of the analytic methods.)
• recommend a daily dosage that would provide a clinically appropriate amount of glucosamine or chondroitin.

MSM

ConsumerLab.com purchased 17 MSM dietary supplements, several of which also contained other ingredients, such as glucosamine, chondroitin, or vitamin C. The products were tested for their labeled amounts of MSM and for contamination with DMSO. The specific tests used to evaluate these products and the standards for passing the tests appear here under "Testing methods" and "Passing score."

TESTING METHODS

Analyses for MSM and DMSO were performed using a gas chromatography (GC) method in an independent laboratory. Products that didn't contain passing levels of MSM or that contained DMSO were retested in a second independent laboratory using a comparable GC method.

Independent laboratories conducted all tests without knowing the identities of the products.

PASSING SCORE

To receive a passing score, a product had to meet these criteria in either a first or second round of testing:
• contain at least 100% but no more than 125% of its labeled amount of MSM
• contain less than 0.05% DMSO (%wt/wt).

Retesting was performed in a second independent laboratory. For a product to fail, confirmation of a failing result on at least one of the parameters above was required on repeat testing.

SAMe

ConsumerLab.com purchased 13 brands of SAMe and tested them for their SAMe levels. The specific tests used to evaluate these products and the standards for passing the tests appear here under "Testing methods" and "Passing score."

TESTING METHODS

SAMe products were tested for their levels of S-adenosyl-methionine (SAMe plus levels of breakdown products). Testing was first conducted in an independent laboratory using high-performance liquid chromatography (HPLC). Because the most appropriate method for testing SAMe products is still under debate, all products were also simultaneously tested for levels of SAMe by a second independent laboratory using a complementary capillary electrophoresis method. Products failing these two tests were reanalyzed by a third independent laboratory using another HPLC method.

The independent laboratories conducted all tests without knowing the identities of the products.

PASSING SCORE

To receive a passing score, a product had to meet these criteria for any of the analytic methods applied:

• meet its claimed weight for free SAMe
• clearly and accurately state the weight of free SAMe (not SAMe plus a stabilizing compound) and not exceed the claimed weight by more than 10%, and total degradation products (combined levels of adenine, S-adenosyl-L-homocysteine and methylthioadenosine) couldn't exceed 10% of the claimed weight for free SAMe.

Retesting took place in a third independent laboratory if a product didn't pass the first two tests.

Saw palmetto

ConsumerLab.com purchased 27 leading brands of saw palmetto and tested them for the quality and quantity of the main ingredient. The specific tests used to evaluate these products and the standards for passing the tests appear here under "Testing methods" and "Passing score."

TESTING METHODS

The chemical constituents of saw palmetto dietary supplement products were analyzed by gas chromatographic analysis for total fatty acids and sterols.

Any product that failed the test was sent to another independent laboratory for retesting. Independent laboratories conducted all tests without knowing the identities of the products.

PASSING SCORE

To receive a passing score, a product had to meet these criteria in either a first or second round of testing:

- meet or exceed its label claims for saw palmetto
- suggest a daily dosage for a clinically appropriate amount of saw palmetto berry extract or saw palmetto berry
- meet or exceed the minimum percentage for weight regarding total and individual fatty acid and sterol components (see Expected fatty acids and sterols, page 149.)

Soy & red clover isoflavones

ConsumerLab.com purchased 18 supplements containing soy or red clover isoflavones. According to their labels, 12 products were made from soy isoflavones, 2 were made from red clover isoflavones, and 4 were made from combinations of soy and red clover isoflavones. The products were tested for their total isoflavone content (specifically glucosidic and aglycone forms of the isoflavones). The specific tests used to evaluate these products and the standards for passing the tests appear here under "Testing methods" and "Passing score."

TESTING METHODS

All products were analyzed using a high-performance liquid chromatography (HPCL) assay in an independent laboratory. The extraction and HPLC method was designed to specifically test for the presence and amount of various glycosidic and aglycone forms of the isoflavones found in soy and red clover.

Products not passing the initial assay were retested in a second laboratory using a similar HPLC assay. Independent laboratories conducted all tests without knowing the identities of the products.

PASSING SCORE

To receive a passing score, a product had to meet these criteria in either a first or second round of testing:

- meet 100% of its label claim for total isoflavone content and, if declared, for specific glucosidic or aglycone isoflavones. (Total isoflavones were calculated as the sum of the glucosidic and aglycone forms.)

St. John's wort

ConsumerLab.com purchased 21 brands of St. John's wort products; 18 claimed to contain standardized extracts, and the remaining 3 claimed to be combinations of extract and raw herb. All but 3 products made claims about hypericin content, and 2 products made claims for both hypericin and hyperforin content. All but 4 of the 21 products also identified the portion of the St. John's wort plant used, such as the flower, flower and leaves, or aerial portions. The products were tested for total hypericin, total hyperforin (if claimed), and contamination with the heavy metal, cadmium. The specific tests used to evaluate these products and the standards for passing the tests appear here under "Testing methods" and "Passing score."

TESTING METHODS

All products were first analyzed for total hypericin using both the Deutscher Arzneimittel-Codex 1986 method (DAC '86) and separate high-performance liquid chromatography (HPLC) methods. The same tests were used to test for hyperforin. Products that failed were then retested using the 1991 UV/Vis spectroscopic method (DAC '91 recalculated to DAC '86) as well as by HPLC methods developed by the Institute for Nutraceutical Advancement's Method Validation Program to specifically test for the presence and amount of hyperforin, hypericin, and pseudohypericin.

Analyses for cadmium were made using atomic absorption with a graphite furnace and inductively coupled plasma/mass spectroscopy.

Any product that didn't pass testing was sent to another independent laboratory to repeat testing for at least one of the failing criteria. Independent laboratories conducted all tests without knowing the identities of the products.

PASSING SCORE

To receive a passing score, a product had to meet these criteria in either a first or second round of testing:

• contain its labeled amount for total hypericin and total hyperforin, with a minimum of 0.3% total hypericin, which is the industry standard (If hypericin or hyperforin levels weren't clearly labeled, ConsumerLab.com set specific minimum standards consistent with most St. John's wort clinical research and tested for those amounts.)

• contain less than 0.3 parts per million (or micrograms per gram) of cadmium for dried raw herb (World Health Organization, Quality Control Methods for Medicinal Plant Material, proposed guidelines, 1998) or less than 0.1 parts per million for extracts. (The concentration standard for extracts results is lower than that for dried herbs because heavy metals, such as cadmium, are partially removed during the extraction process.)

Valerian

ConsumerLab.com purchased 17 valerian products: 7 valerian extracts, 6 valerian powders, and 4 combinations of the 2. Although most products stated that they contained only valerian, 5 listed one or more additional herbs, such as kava kava, hops, lemon balm, and skullcap. All had adequate labeling indicating the proper species and plant part as well as the valerian amount, and 8 also claimed to be standardized to provide specific levels of valerenic acids. The products were tested for their valerenic acid content. The specific tests used to evaluate these products and the standards for passing the tests appear here under "Testing methods" and "Passing score."

TESTING METHODS

Valerian products were tested for acetoxyvalerenic acid, hydroxyvalerenic acid, valerenic acid, and valernal. All products were first analyzed for the valerenic acid constituents using a high-performance liquid chromatography (HPLC) assay in an independent laboratory. This HPLC method was developed by the Institute for Nutraceutical Advancement's Method Validation Program to specifically test for the presence and amount of acetoxyvalerenic acid, hydroxyvalerenic acid, valerenic acid, and valernal.

Products not passing the initial assay were retested in a second independent laboratory using a similar HPLC assay. Independent laboratories conducted all tests without knowing the identities of the products.

PASSING SCORE

To receive a passing score, a product had to meet these criteria in either a first or second round of testing:

• Clearly and accurately provide all of the label information required by the U.S. Food and Drug Administration—

Species of valerian used (Valerian; V. officinalis L.)

Part of the plant used (root or rhizome)

Form of valerian used (root powder, extract, or tincture)

Amount of valerian per pill or dose in grams or milligrams (1 gram = 1,000 mg)

• meet its label claims for total valerenic acid content, with a minimum of 0.17% total valerenic acids for root powder preparations, more for extracts. (Because there may be a slight loss of ingredient during the extraction process, 3X to 6X extracts or tinctures [or 3:1 to 6:1, respectively] were expected to have a minimum for total valerenic acids of 0.4% to 0.8%, respectively. Total valerenic acids were calculated as the sum of acetoxyvalerenic acid and valerenic acid. Hydroxyvalerenic acid wasn't included in this calculation because it may be a degradation product rather than an inherent marker compound.)

More brand information

Here are the web addresses and phone numbers for the manufacturers and distributors of each brand listed as "approved quality" in the product reviews. (Review(s) in which the product(s) are listed appear below in italics.) Some brands include additional product information provided by the manufacturer or distributor and is considered advertising. This information was current when the book went to press but may change anytime.

AARP
Multivitamins & multiminerals
AARP
www.aarppharmacy.com
800-456-2277

Action Labs
MSM
Nutraceutical Corp.
www.nutraceutical.com
800-579-4665

Aflexa
Glucosamine & chondroitin
McNeil Consumer Healthcare
www.aflexa.com
800-243-5822

ARTHxDS
Glucosamine & chondroitin
Medtech, Inc.
www.arthx.com
800-443-4908

Body Fortress
Creatine
U.S. Nutritionals
www.naturesbounty.com
800-433-2990

Brite-Life
Vitamin E
Bergen Brunswig Drug Company
714-385-4000

Cal Burst®
Calcium
Pharmavite Corporation
www.naturemade.com
800-276-2878

Caltrate®
Calcium
Wyeth Consumer Healthcare
www.caltrate.com
800-282-8805
Products Sold: Total of six types of CALTRATE: regular, +D, Plus, +Soy, Chewable Plus and

Colon Health in various tablet counts.
Where to Buy: Most food, drug, mass
merchandise, and warehouse club stores
nationwide.

CALTRATE® 600 Plus (Listed in "Calcium")
CALTRATE Plus provides 600 mg of elemental
calcium from calcium carbonate, vitamin D for
absorption, and selected other minerals
important for bone health. Take with or
without a multivitamin.

Carlson

CoQ10, Vitamin E
Carlson, Division of J.R. Carlson
Laboratories
www.carlsonlabs.com
847-255-1600

Celestial Seasonings

Ginseng, Saw palmetto, Valerian
Celestial Seasonings, Inc.
www.celestialseasonings.com
800-351-8175

Centrum®

*Calcium,Ginkgo biloba, Ginseng,
Multivitamins & multiminerals, Saw palmetto,
Vitamin C*
Wyeth Consumer Healthcare
www.centrum.com
877-236-8786
Products Sold: Shamu characters discontinued
in 2000. Same Centrum Kids formulas now
available in RUGRATS® characters (Trademark
of Nickelodeon/Viacom). CENTRUM Kids
RUGRATS® comes in three formulas:
Complete, Extra C, and Extra Calcium.
Where to Buy: Most food, drug, and mass
merchandise stores, and selected warehouse
clubs nationwide.

*CENTRUM® Kids Chewable Vitamin with
Extra C* (Listed in "Vitamin C")

*CENTRUM® Kids Chewable Vitamin with
Extra "Calcium"* (Listed in "Calcium")
Provide complete supplemental nutrition that
mother's demand in the appealing RUGRATS®

characters that kids love to take.

CENTRUM® Silver (Listed in "Multivitamins
& multiminerals")
Complete multivitamin specially formulated in
accordance with the FDA–set Daily Values for
adults ages 50+. Contains no iron; more
calcium, chromium, and vitamins B_6, B_{12}, and
E; and less vitamin K and phosphorous vs.
CENTRUM® complete multivitamin for adults
younger than age 50. Offered in 60 ct, 100 ct,
150 ct, and 300 ct (that is, two 150-ct bottles
shrink-wrapped together).

Citracal

Calcium
Mission Pharmacal
www.citracal.com
800-531-3333

Cosamin® DS

Glucosamine & chondroitin
Nutramax Laboratories, Inc.
www.nutramaxlabs.com
www.cosamin.com
800-925-5187
Products Sold: Nutraceuticals for the consumer
and veterinary market—Cosamin®DS, Senior
Moment®, CoMax Q10®, Biosel®,
Cosequin®, Denosyl® SD4
Where to Buy: Food, drug, mass merchandise,
and health food stores as well as over the
internet.

Cosamin® DS (Listed in "Glucosamine &
chondroitin")
Even though labels appear to be the same,
published research shows that
glucosamine/chondroitin sulfate brands are
not the same. CosaminDS is the only
glucosamine/chondroitin sulfate brand proven
effective in controlled clinical studies
conducted and published in the United States.
The identical chondroitin sulfate used
exclusively in CosaminDS was selected by the
National Institutes of Health for a major clinical
study. CosaminDS is the #1 doctor-and-
pharmacist-recommended brand.

More brand information

Country Life
Ginkgo biloba, Iron
Country Life
www.country-life.com
800-645-5768

Cowboy Smart
MSM
John Ewing Comp.
www.johnewing.com
800-525-8601

CVS
CoQ10, Echinacea, Ginkgo biloba,
Glucosamine & chondroitin, MSM,
Saw palmetto, Vitamin C
CVS
www.cvs.com
800-746-7287

Doctor's Best
MSM
Doctor's Best, Inc.
www.doctorsbest.net
800-333-6977

Drugstore.com
Vitamin E
Drugstore.com
www.drugstore.com
800-378-4786

EAS
Creatine
EAS
www.eas.com
800-297-9776

Eckerd
Valerian
Eckerd Drug Company
www.eckerd.com
800-325-3737

Enzymatic Therapy
Ginkgo biloba, Glucosamine & chondroitin,
Saw palmetto, St. John's wort
Enzymatic Therapy
www.enzy.com
800-558-7372

Feosol
Iron
GlaxoSmithKline Consumer Healthcare
www.feosol.com
800-897-7535

Fergon
Iron
Bayer
www.bayercare.com
800-331-4536

Ferro-Sequels
Iron
Inverness Medical, Inc.
www.invernessmedical.com
800-899-7353

Fields of Nature
Calcium, CoQ10, Glucosamine & chondroitin
IVC Industries, Inc.
www.ivcinc.com
800-666-8482

Flex-A-Min®
Glucosamine & chondroitin, MSM
Arthritis Research Corp.
www.flexamin.com
800-255-8490

Flintstones
Calcium, Multivitamins & multiminerals
Bayer
www.bayercare.com
800-331-4536

Frontier
Echinacea
Frontier
www.frontierherb.com
800-786-1388

Gary Null
CoQ10
Gary Null & Associates
www.garynull.com
646-505-4660

Geritol
Multivitamins & multiminerals
GlaxoSmithKline Consumer Healthcare
www.geritol.com
800-897-7535

Ginkai
Ginkgo biloba
Lichtwer Pharma
www.lichtwer.com
732-389-9100

Ginkoba
Ginkgo biloba
Pharmaton Natural Health Products
www.ginkoba.com
800-451-6688

Ginsana
Ginseng
Pharmaton Natural Health Products
www.ginsana.com
800-451-6688

GNC
Calcium, CoQ10, Ginkgo biloba, Glucosamine & chondroitin, SAMe, Saw palmetto, Soy & red clover isoflavones
GNC
www.gnc.com
888-462-2548

Good Neighbor
Iron
Bergen Brunswig Drug Company
www.mygnp.com
714-385-4000

Harmonex
St. John's wort
Chattem
www.chattem.com
800-366-6833

Health From the Sun
Fish oils: Omega-3 fatty acids (EPA & DHA)
Health From the Sun
www.healthfromthesun.com
800-447-2229

Health Pride
Echinacea
Farmer Jack/Compass Foods
www.farmerjack.com
877-327-5225

Health Smart Vitamins
St. John's wort
HealthSmart Vitamins
www.healthsmartvitamins.com
800-492-3003

Healthy Woman
Soy & red clover isoflavones
McNeil Consumer Healthcare
www.jnj.com
800-962-5357

Herbalife
St. John's wort
Herbalife
www.herbalife.com
310-216-9661

More brand information

Jarrow Formulas
Fish oils: Omega-3 fatty acids (EPA & DHA), MSM
Jarrow Formulas, Inc.
www.jarrow.com
800-726-0886

Kal
Vitamin E
Nutraceutical Corp.
www.nutraceutical.com
800-579-4665

Kira
St. John's wort
Lichtwer Pharma
www.lichtwer.com
732-389-9100

Kirkland
Multivitamins & multiminerals, Vitamin C, Vitamin E
Costco/CWC
www.costco.com
800-774-2678

Kroger
Vitamin E
The Kroger Co.
www.kroger.com
866-221-4141

Life Extension
Vitamin E
Life Extension Foundation
www.lef.org
800-678-8989

Longs
St. John's wort
Longs Drug Stores
www.longs.com
800-421-1168

Maalox
Calcium
Novartis Consumer Health, Inc.
www.novartis.com
800-452-0051

Marquee
B Vitamins
Fleming Companies, Inc.
www.fleming.com
972-906-8000

Mason
B Vitamins
Mason Vitamins, Inc.
www.masonvitamins.com
800-327-6005

Medicine Shoppe Vitamin
B Vitamins
Medicine Shoppe International, Inc.
www.medicineshoppe.com
800-325-1397

Meijer
Vitamin E
Meijer, Inc.
www.meijer.com
616-453-6711

Member's Mark
Fish oils: Omega-3 fatty acids (EPA & DHA)
SWC (Sam's Club)
www.samsclub.com
888-746-7726

MET-Rx® Engineered Nutrition
Creatine
MET-Rx USA
www.metrx.com
800-556-3879

Minute Maid
Calcium
The Minute Maid Company
www.minutemaid.com
888-884-8952

Mother Nature.com
Ginkgo biloba, Saw palmetto
Mother Nature, Inc.
www.mothernature.com
800-439-5506

Movana
St. John's wort
Pharmaton Natural Health Products
www.pharmaton.com
800-451-6688

Muscletech
Creatine
MuscleTech Research and
Development Inc.
www.muscletech.com
888-334-4448

Mylanta
Calcium
Johnson & Johnson/Merck
www.mylanta.com
800-469-5268

Natrol
*CoQ10, Creatine, Ginkgo biloba,
Glucosamine & chondroitin, SAMe,
Saw palmetto, Vitamin C*
Natrol, Inc.
www.natrol.com
800-326-1520

Natural Balance
MSM
Natural Balance, Inc.
www.naturalbalance.com
800-833-8737

Natural Factors
Vitamin E
Natural Factors Nutritional Products Ltd.
www.naturalfactors.com
800-322-8704

Natural Wealth
Vitamin C
Natural Wealth Nutrition Corp.
516-244-2055

NaturaLife
Echinacea, Ginseng
NaturaLife Corp.
800-531-3233

Naturally Kids
Vitamin C
Naturally Vitamins
www.naturallyvitamins.com
800-899-4499

Naturally Preferred
Echinacea
Inter-American Products, Inc.
www.kroger.com
800-632-6900

Naturally Vitamins
Calcium
Naturally Vitamins
www.naturallyvitamins.com
800-899-4499

Nature Made®
*B Vitamins, Calcium, CoQ10, Ginkgo biloba,
Ginseng, Glucosamine & chondroitin, Iron,
MSM, Multivitamins & multiminerals, SAMe,
Soy & red clover isoflavones, St. John's wort,
Vitamin C, Vitamin E*
Pharmavite Corp.
www.NatureMade.com
800-276-2878
Products Sold: Pharmavite manufactures
Nature Made vitamins, Nature's Resource

More brand information

herbs and other supplements designed to promote health. Where to Buy: Food, drug, and mass merchandise stores. Visit NatureMade.com for specific information on where to buy.

Balanced B-150 B-Complex—Timed Release (Listed in "B Vitamins")
Nature Made B-150 is a combination of essential B vitamins: thiamine, riboflavin, niacin, vitamin B_6, and pantothenic acid. The B vitamins are involved in the body's energy production and help to maintain the health of the heart, nerves, skin, eyes, hair, liver, and mouth. Visit NatureMade.com for more information on ingredients, precautions, and proper dosage.

CalBurst Calcium Supplement (Chocolate & Creamy Vanilla) (Listed in "Calcium")
CalBurst Calcium supplements deliver half the daily requirements of calcium and vitamin D in a great-tasting soft chew. Calcium supplementation is a key factor in building and maintaining bones and helping sustain a healthy nervous system. Health professionals recommend calcium supplements that contain Vitamin D, which stimulates the absorption of calcium. Visit NatureMade.com for more information on ingredients, precautions, and proper dosage.

Calcium and Magnesium with Zinc (Listed in "Calcium")
Nature Made Calcium/Magnesium/Zinc provides three important minerals in one daily dose. Calcium is key in building and maintaining bones and helping sustain a healthy nervous system. Magnesium is important in bone health and helps regulate calcium metabolism. Zinc, essential for healthy immune function, is required in the body for growth and development. Visit Nature-Made.com for more information on ingredients, precautions, and proper dosage.

CoQ-10 (100 mg) (Listed in "CoQ10")
Coenzyme Q10 occurs in the cells of all plants and animals, but dietary sources do not provide adequate levels of this nutrient. CoQ-10 is an important fat-soluble antioxidant that protects the body's cells from free radical damage. CoQ-10 is necessary for the production of energy in all cells of the body and may also play a role in heart health. Visit NatureMade.com for more information on ingredients, precautions, and proper dosage.

Essential Balance (Listed in "Multivitamins & multiminerals")
Nature Made Essential Balance provides a balance of 13 key vitamins and 18 minerals essential each day to support a healthy lifestyle. Taking a high-quality multivitamin and multimineral serves as the foundation of a nutritional supplementation program. Visit NatureMade.com for more information on ingredients, precautions, and proper dosage.

Ginkgo biloba 40 mg (Listed in "Ginkgo biloba")
Nature Made Ginkgo Biloba helps maintain mental alertness, concentration, and memory. Studies indicate that ginkgo biloba may increase peripheral circulation, thereby enhancing blood flow to the arms, legs, and brain. Visit NatureMade.com for more information on ingredients, precautions, and proper dosage.

Glucosamine 500 mg (Listed in "Glucosamine & chondroitin")
Glucosamine is produced naturally in the body and plays a role in proper joint function and joint flexibility. Supplementing the diet with glucosamine stimulates the formation of cartilage, promoting joint comfort and flexibility. Nature Made Glucosamine 500 mg provides more glucosamine than many competitive products and contains no sodium. Visit NatureMade.com for more information on ingredients, precautions, and proper dosage.

Iron 65 mg (Listed in "Iron")
Iron is necessary to prevent iron-deficiency anemia, a condition in which red blood cells cannot carry enough oxygen to meet the body's needs, which leads to fatigue and poor concentration; this condition affects 20% of women and 3% of men. Iron also helps strengthen the immune system and aids in

the manufacturing of collagen, a protein that builds connective tissues. Visit Nature-Made.com for more information on ingredients, precautions, and proper dosage.

Joint Action (Listed in "Glucosamine & chondroitin," "SAMe")
Nature Made Joint Action contains SAMe and glucosamine, two naturally occurring compounds contributing to joint health. SAMe is critical in the manufacture and maintenance of cartilage, whereas glucosamine may help repair and maintain cartilage and stimulate cartilage cell growth. Visit NatureMade.com for more information on ingredients, precautions, and proper dosage.

SAM-e 200 mg (tosylate) (Listed in "SAMe")
SAM-e, short for S-adensylmethionine, is "your body's own mood enhancer." It is involved in several biological reactions in the human body and is clinically proven to support emotional well-being. Nature Made was the first brand to market SAM-e in the United States and continues to support ongoing clinical research to support its validity and varied uses. Visit NatureMade.com for more information on ingredients, precautions, and proper dosage.

Soy50 Menopause Supplement (Listed in "Soy & red clover isoflavones")
Scientific studies have shown that soy may have a beneficial effect on women's health as they grow older. By exerting weak estrogen-like activity, soy isoflavones offer some of the same benefits as human estrogen. Soy isoflavones may help reduce hot flashes and night sweats associated with menopause. Visit NatureMade.com for more information on ingredients, precautions, and proper dosage.

St. John's wort 300 mg extract (Listed in "St. John's wort")
Nature Made St. John's wort may help enhance mood and emotional well-being. More than 30 clinical studies show that St. John's wort is effective in helping improve mood. Visit NatureMade.com for more information on ingredients, precautions, and proper dosage.

Triple Flex (Listed in "Glucosamine & chondroitin," "MSM")
Nature Made Triple Flex offers the triple action of glucosamine, chondroitin, and MSM. These three components work together to support joint health and mobility, contributing to a healthy and active lifestyle. Visit NatureMade.com for more information on ingredients, precautions, and proper dosage.

Vitamin C 1,000 mg (Listed in "Vitamin C")
Vitamin C is a powerful antioxidant, essential for proper immune function. It helps the body manufacture collagen, a key protein in our connective tissues, cartilage, and tendons. Vitamin C also aids in the absorption and utilization of other nutrients, such as vitamin E and iron. Visit NatureMade.com for more information on ingredients, precautions, and proper dosage.

Vitamin E 400 I.U. (Listed in "Vitamin E")
Vitamin E is a powerful antioxidant that helps boost the immune system and maintain red blood cells and muscle tissues. Many scientific studies support vitamin E's role in maintaining heart health. Because of vitamin E's strong antioxidant effects, supplementation provides a protective effect in many common health conditions. Visit NatureMade.com for more information on ingredients, precautions, and proper dosage.

Nature's Best
Creatine
Nature's Best
www.naturesbest.com
800-345-2378

Nature's Bounty®
B Vitamins, Calcium, CoQ10, Echinacea, Ginkgo biloba, Glucosamine & chondroitin, Iron, MSM, Multivitamins & multiminerals, St. John's wort, Vitamin C, Vitamin E
Nature's Bounty, Inc.
www.naturesbounty.com
800-433-2990

More brand information

Nature's Plus
Calcium, CoQ10, MSM, St. John's wort
Natural Organics, Inc.
www.naturesplus.com
631-293-0030

Nature's Resource®
Ginkgo biloba, Soy & red clover isoflavones,
St. John's wort, Valerian
Pharmavite Corporation
www.naturesresource.com
800-423-2405
Products Sold: Full line of herbs: whole herbs,
extracts, and time-release herb products.
Where to Buy: Food, drug, and mass
merchandise stores nationwide.
Ginkgo biloba 60 mg Extract (Listed in
"Ginkgo biloba")
60 mg of ginkgo biloba extract (standardized
to contain 24% flavone glycosides) in a two-
piece capsule. Dosage suggestion: 1 capsule
twice daily. Clinical studies show that ginkgo
biloba (120 mg/day) can be effective in
enhancing cognitive function. No artificial
colors, flavors, or preservatives. Purity, quality,
and satisfaction guaranteed. If you have
questions about Nature's Resource Ginkgo
Biloba, call 1-800-314-HERB.
Soy Isoflavones 50 mg Extract (Listed in "Soy
& red clover isoflavones")
50 mg of soy isoflavones extract in a two-
piece capsule. Dosage suggestion: 1 to
2 capsules/day. Studies show that isoflavones
(50 to 90 mg/day), the active components of
soy, may help maintain bone health and
support a woman's body during menopause.
No artificial colors, flavors, or preservatives.
Purity, quality, and satisfaction guaranteed. If
you have questions about Nature's Resource
Soy, call 1-800-314-HERB.
St. John's wort 300 mg Extract (Listed in "St.
John's wort")
300 mg of St. John's wort extract
(standardized to contain 0.3% hypericin by
UV) in a two-piece capsule. Dosage
suggestion: 1 capsule three times daily. Clinical

studies show that St. John's wort (300 mg
three times daily) can be effective for mood
enhancement. NO artificial colors, flavors, or
preservatives. Purity, quality, and satisfaction
guaranteed. If you have questions about
Nature's Resource St. Johns' Wort, call 1-800-
314-HERB.
Valerian 100 mg Extract (Listed in
"Valerian")
100 mg of valerian extract in a softgel form.
Dosage suggestion: 1 or 2 softgels 1 hour
before bedtime. Clinical research shows that
valerian may help promote sleep. No artificial
colors, flavor, or preservatives. Purity, quality,
and satisfaction guaranteed. If you have
questions about Nature's Resource Valerian,
call 1-800-314-HERB.

Nature's Sunshine
Multivitamins & multiminerals
Nature's Sunshine Products, Inc.
www.naturessunshine.com
800-223-8225

Nature's Valley
B Vitamins
American Procurement & Logistics
Company
800-405-7787

Nature's Way
CoQ10, Echinacea, Fish oils: Omega-3 fatty
acids (EPA & DHA), Ginkgo biloba, Saw
palmetto, Vitamin C, Vitamin E
Nature's Way Products, Inc.
www.naturesway.com
800-926-8883

Naturvite Natural Vitamins
B Vitamins
Solgar Vitamin and Herb
www.solgar.com
877-765-4274

NOW®

CoQ10, Ginkgo biloba, Glucosamine & chondroitin, MSM
NOW Foods
www.nowfoods.com
630-545-9098

NutraLife

SAMe
NutraLife Health Products
www.nutralife.com
877-688-7254

Nutrilite®

Calcium, CoQ10, Echinacea, Fish oils: Omega-3 fatty acids (EPA & DHA), Ginkgo biloba, Glucosamine & chondroitin, Iron,‗ Multivitamins & multiminerals, Saw palmetto, Soy & red clover isoflavones, St. John's wort, Valerian, Vitamin C, Vitamin E
Access Business Group International
www.nutrilite.com
www.quixtar.com
800-253-6500

Products Sold: Nutrilite is a leading global brand of vitamins, minerals, and dietary supplements as well as food products.

Where to Buy: Nutrilite is available only through Quixtar Independent Business Owners. Call 1-800-544-7167.

Bio C Plus (Listed in "Vitamin C")
Fight free radicals and support your immune system with this exclusive vitamin C formula. Acerola cherries have more vitamin C per ounce than oranges—and this formula includes natural acerola cherry concentrate (30 mg), citrus bioflavonoid concentrate from lemon pulp and peel (35 mg), and other rich sources to supply 250 mg of vitamin C per tablet. 300 tablets.

Black Cohosh and Soy (Listed in "Soy & red clover isoflavones")
Get two to four times the black cohosh of leading brands, plus calcium, soy protein, and isoflavones for a broad range of benefits. Black cohosh and soy have both been shown to relieve menopause symptoms, especially when

taken over time. A daily serving (3 tablets) contains 120 mg of black cohosh extract, 300 mg of soy protein, 49.8 mg of isoflavones, 30 mg of acerola cherry concentrate, and 60 mg of calcium. 90 tablets.

Calcium Magnesium Plus (Listed in "Calcium")
The Daily Value for calcium is 900 mg, but most adults get only 400 mg in their diet. With 3 tablets/day of this formula, you get the bone-building benefits of 650 mg of calcium and 325 mg of magnesium, plus 10 mg of zinc, 2 mg of copper, 2.5 mg of manganese, and phytonutrients from alfalfa. 250 tablets.

CoEnzyme Q10 (Listed in "CoQ10")
As we age, our bodies may not produce enough CoQ10—an important "spark plug" nutrient. Each capsule gives you 30 mg of CoQ10 for heart and liver support; 100 mg of L-carnitine, an amino acid essential for fat metabolism; 125 mg of taurine to help maintain biochemical reactions involved in muscle contraction; and beneficial phytonutrients from Nutrilite Bioflavonoid Complex. 60 capsules.

Daily Multivitamin Multimineral Supplement (Listed in "Multivitamins & multiminerals")
Just 1 tablet/day gives you 100% or more of the Daily Value for 24 vitamins and minerals. The exclusive alfalfa/watercress/parsley and acerola concentrates provide important plant-based nutrients over and above vitamins and minerals. It's the easy way to get the nutrients you need each day. 180 tablets.

Double X® Vitamin Mineral Phytonutrient Supplement (Listed in "Multivitamins & multiminerals")
The multi for energy you can feel, all day. It fills the gaps in your diet with 45 vitamins, minerals, and plant concentrates, many from natural sources grown on Nutrilite's certified-organic farms. A clinical study shows that people who use Double X have higher blood levels of many essential nutrients than those who eat an optimal diet averaging 7.8 servings of fruits and vegetables a day. 31-day supply.

More brand information

Ginkgo biloba and DHA (Listed in "Ginkgo biloba")
This powerhouse herbal gives you what you need to help keep your brain healthy. Just 3 tablets/day delivers 160 mg of standardized ginkgo biloba extract for mental acuity, 180 mg of DHA (an important omega-3 fatty acid) for overall brain health and development, and 68 mg of gotu kola, which herbalists believe helps energize the brain. 100 softgels.

Glucosamine HCl with Boswellia (Listed in "Glucosamine & chondroitin")
This powerhouse herbal gives you what you need to help keep your brain healthy. Three tablets a day deliver 160 mg standardized ginkgo biloba extract for mental acuity, 180 mg DHA – an important omega-3 fatty acid – for overall brain health and development, and 68 mg gotu kola, which herbalists believe helps energize the brain. 100 softgels.

Iron-Folic Plus (Listed in "Iron")
The FDA has stated that getting enough iron and folic acid early in pregnancy may help prevent neural-tube birth defects. Each tablet provides 33% of the Daily Value of folic acid, and 83% of the iron a woman's body needs— especially during pregnancy. If there's a chance you may become pregnant, consider Iron-Folic Plus as a dietary supplement. Think of it as preventive care for baby and you. 120 tablets. Certified Kosher.

Omega-3 Complex (Listed in "Fish oils: Omega-3 fatty acids [EPA & DHA]")
Omega-3 fatty acids support normal heart health and cholesterol levels. If you aren't meeting your daily needs by eating fish like salmon and tuna, try nature's richest source of alpha linolenic acid—flaxseed oil. Omega 3 Complex softgels contain a unique blend of 185 mg of alpha linolenic acid, plus 65 mg of EPA, 45 mg of DHA , and 30 I.U. (100% Daily Value) of vitamin E. For fish benefits without the fishy taste. 90 softgels.

Parselenium-E® (Listed in "Vitamin E")
A natural combination of 400 I.U. of vitamin E and 10 mcg of selenium, nutrients that work together to prevent oxidative damage to the body's cells. Unlike isolated synthetic vitamin E, this formula gives you a full spectrum of natural tocopherols, including d-alpha-tocopherol, a form that is especially stable. Parsley concentrate from plants grown on Nutrilite farms adds phytonutrients. 60 tablets.

St. John's wort with Lemon Balm (Listed in "St. John's wort")
Contains soothing herbs plus vitamins and natural plant nutrients to offer nutritional support for maintaining a healthy mood. Each capsule contains 300 mg of St. John's wort (standardized to contain 0.3% hypericin) plus 26 mg of lemon balm, 24 mg of citrus bioflavonoid concentrate, and 10 mg of acerola cherry concentrate. 90 capsules.

Triple Guard Echinacea (Listed in "Echinacea")
Nutrilite grows all the echinacea used in its tablet, liquid and spray echinacea products on certified-organic Trout Lake Farm, controlling purity and potency from seed to supplement. Three extracts are used for the broadest spectrum of echinacea coverage: *Echinacea angustifolia* root extract and *E. purpurea* aerial parts extract and root extract. Also contains citrus bioflavonoid complex (100 mg). 120 tablets, 168 mg of echinacea blend per tablet.

Valerian and Hops (Listed in "Valerian")
Valerenic acid has been clinically proven to help people fall asleep faster and stay asleep longer. This safe, natural, proprietary blend contains 450 mg of valerian extract per 3-tablet serving, standardized to contain 0.8% valerenic acid, plus 150 mg of whole valerian root extract, 100 mg of hops extract, and 150 mg of lemon balm extract. 90 tablets.

Nutrition Now
Echinacea
Nutrition Now
www.nutritionnow.com
800-929-0418

Ocuvite
Multivitamins & multiminerals
Bausch & Lomb
www.bausch.com
800-553-5340

One-A-Day
Calcium, Ginkgo biloba, Ginseng,
Glucosamine & chondroitin, Multivitamins &
multiminerals, Saw palmetto, St. John's wort,
Vitamin C
Bayer
www.oneaday.com
800-331-4536

Optimum Nutrition
Echinacea
Optimum Nutrition
www.optimumnutrition.com
630-236-0097

Os Cal
Calcium
GlaxoSmithKline Consumer Healthcare
www.oscal.com
800-897-7535

Osteo Bi-Flex®
Glucosamine & chondroitin
Rexall Sundown, Inc.
www.osteobiflex.com
888-848-2435

Perfect Choice
B Vitamins
Inter-American Products, Inc.
www.kroger.com
800-632-6900

Pharmanex
Multivitamins & multiminerals, Valerian
Pharmanex
www.pharmanex.com
800-487-1000

PharmAssure
Ginseng, Saw palmetto, Vitamin E
PharmAssure/Rite Aid Corporation
www.riteaid.com
800-748-3243

PhytoPharmica
Ginkgo biloba, Glucosamine & chondroitin,
Saw palmetto
PhytoPharmica
www.PhytoPharmica.com
800-553-2370

Planetary Formulas
Valerian
Planetary Formulas
www.planetaryformulas.com
800-606-6226

PlanetRx
MSM
PlanetRx.com, Inc.
Discontinued

Poly-Vi-Sol
Multivitamins & multiminerals
Mead Johnson Nutritionals
www.enfamil.com
800-222-9123

Posture-D
Calcium
Inverness Medical, Inc.
www.invernessmedical.com
800-899-7353

Precision Engineered
Creatine
U.S. Nutritionals
www.vitaminworld.com
631-244-2125

More brand information

Prolab
Creatine
Prolab
www.prolab.com
800-326-1520

Promensil
Soy & red clover isoflavones
Novogen
www.promensil.com
877-417-7663

Propalmex
Saw palmetto
Chattem
www.chattem.com
800-366-6833

Pure Encapsulations
Fish oils: Omega-3 fatty acids (EPA & DHA)
Pure Encapsulations, Inc.
www.purecaps.com
800-753-2277

Puritan's Pride®
B Vitamins, Calcium, CoQ10, Echinacea, Fish oils: Omega-3 fatty acids (EPA & DHA), Ginkgo biloba, Glucosamine & chondroitin, Iron, Multivitamins & multiminerals, SAMe, Saw palmetto, Vitamin C, Vitamin E
Puritan's Pride, Inc.
www.puritan.com
800-645-1030

Q-Gel
CoQ10
Gel-Tec, Div. of Tishcon
www.tishcon.com
800-848-8442

Quanterra
Ginkgo biloba, Saw palmetto
Warner-Lambert Company
Brand Discontinued

Ricola
Valerian
Ricola
www.ricola.com
973-984-6811

Rolaids
Calcium
Warner-Lambert Company
www.acidrelief.com
800-223-0182

Root to Health
Ginseng
Hsu's Ginseng Enterprises, Inc.
www.hsuginseng.com
800-388-3818

Safeway
Iron, Multivitamins & multiminerals, Soy & red clover isoflavones
Safeway
www.safeway.com
877-723-3929

Sav-on
B Vitamins
American Procurement & Logistics Company
www.sav-ondrugs.com
888-746-7252

Schiff
Calcium, CoQ10, Glucosamine & chondroitin, Vitamin C, Vitamin E
Weider Nutritional International
www.schiffvitamins.com
800-526-6251

Sedonium
Valerian
Lichtwer Pharma
www.lichtwer.com
732-389-9100

Sesame Street
Vitamin C
McNeil Consumer Healthcare
800-469-5268

Shaklee
Calcium, Fish oils: Omega-3 fatty acids, Ginkgo biloba, Glucosamine & chondroitin, Saw palmetto, Soy & red clover isoflavones, Vitamin C, Vitamin E
Shaklee
www.shaklee.com
800-742-5533

Shop Rite
Vitamin E
Wakefern Food Corp.
www.shoprite.com
800-746-7748

Slo Niacin
B Vitamins
Upsher-Smith Laboratories, Inc.
www.upsher-smith.com
800-654-2299

Slow Fe
Iron
Novartis Consumer Health, Inc.
www.novartis.com
800-452-0051

Solaray
CoQ10, Iron
Nutraceutical Corp.
www.nutraceutical.com
800-579-4665

Solgar
CoQ10, Fish oils: Omega-3 fatty acids (EPA & DHA), Vitamin E
Solgar Vitamin and Herb
www.solgar.com
877-765-4274

Source Naturals
CoQ10, Creatine, SAMe
Source Naturals, Inc.
www.sourcenaturals.com
800-815-2333

Soy Care
Soy & red clover isoflavones
Inverness Medical, Inc.
www.invernessmedical.com
800-899-7353

Spectrum Essentials
Fish oils: Omega-3 fatty acids (EPA & DHA)
Spectrum Organic Products, Inc.
www.spectrumnaturals.com
707-778-8900

Sport Pharma
Creatine
Sport Pharma USA, Inc.
www.sportpharma.com
800-654-4246

Spring Valley
Calcium, Ginkgo biloba, Glucosamine & chondroitin, MSM, Multivitamins & multiminerals, Saw palmetto, Soy & red clover isoflavones, Vitamin C
Wal-Mart
www.walmart.com
479-273-4000

Stresstabs
B Vitamins
Inverness Medical, Inc.
www.invernessmedical.com
800-899-7353

Stuart Prenatal
Multivitamins & multiminerals
Integrity Pharmaceutical
www.integritypharma.com
800-823-6878

More brand information

Sundown®
Calcium, CoQ10, Ginkgo biloba, Iron,
Multivitamins & multiminerals, Saw palmetto,
Soy & red clover isoflavones, St. John's wort
Rexall Sundown, Inc.
www.sundownnutrition.com

Sunkist
Vitamin C
Novartis Consumer Health, Inc.
www.novartis.com
800-452-0051

Super G
B Vitamins
Giant Food Inc.
www.giantfood.com
888-469-4426

Swanson
Valerian
Swanson Health Products
www.swansonvitamins.com
800-603-3198

Target
B Vitamins, Echinacea
Target Corporation
www.target.com
800-440-0680

The Vitamin Shoppe
CoQ10, Fish oils: Omega-3 fatty acids
(EPA & DHA), SAMe
The Vitamin Shoppe
www.vitaminshoppe.com
888-880-3055

Theragran-M
Multivitamins & multiminerals
Bristol Myers Products
no web site
800-468-7746

Thompson
Ginkgo biloba, Vitamin C
Nutraceutical Corp.
www.nutraceutical.com
800-579-4665

Thorne Research
B Vitamins
Thorne Research, Inc. (Julian Whittaker)
www.thorne.com
208-263-1337

Tom's of Maine
Echinacea
Tom's of Maine, Inc.
www.tomsofmaine.com
800-367-8667

Trader Darwin's
Fish oils: Omega-3 fatty acids (EPA & DHA),
Vitamin E
Trader Joe's
www.traderjoes.com
781-433-0234

Tropicana
Calcium
Tropicana Products, Inc.
www.tropicana.com
800-237-7799

TruNature
CoQ10
Leiner Health Products, Inc.
www.yourlifevitamins.com
800-533-8482

Tums
Calcium
GlaxoSmithKline Consumer Healthcare
www.tums.com
800-897-7535

TwinLab

B Vitamins, CoQ10, Creatine, Echinacea, Fish oils: Omega-3 fatty acids (EPA & DHA), Iron, SAMe, Vitamin E
Twin Laboratories
www.twinlab.com
800-645-5626

Universal Nutrition

Creatine
Universal Nutrition
www.universalnutrition.com
800-872-0101

USANA

Soy & red clover isoflavones, Vitamin E
USANA
www.usana.com
888-950-9595

Viactiv

Calcium
Mead Johnson Nutritionals
www.viactiv.com
877-842-2843

Vitamin World®

B Vitamins, CoQ10, Fish oils: Omega-3 fatty acids (EPA & DHA), Iron, MSM, Multivitamins & multiminerals, Soy & red clover isoflavones, St. John's wort
Vitamin World, Inc.
www.vitaminworld.com
631-244-2125

Vitamins.com

Vitamin E
www.Vitamins.com
Brand Discontinued

VitaSmart

Calcium, iron, Multivitamins & multiminerals, Soy & red clover isoflavones, Vitamin E
Kmart
www.bluelight.com
866-562-7848

Wakunaga

Ginkgo biloba
Wakunaga of America
www.wakunaga.com
800-421-2998

Walgreens

Calcium, Ginkgo biloba, Ginseng, Glucosamine & chondroitin, Multivitamins & multiminerals, Saw palmetto, Vitamin C
Walgreens
www.walgreens.com
800-289-2273

Weider

Creatine
Weider Nutritional International
800-526-6251

Whole Food

Iron, Vitamin C
Whole Foods Market
www.wholefoodsmarket .com
512-477-4455

Windmill

Vitamin C, Vitamin E
Windmill Vitamin Co, Inc.
www.windmillvitamins.com
800-822-4320

Yerba Prima

St. John's wort
Yerba Prima
www.yerbaprima.com
800-488-4339

Your Life

Calcium, CoQ10, Ginkgo biloba, Glucosamine & chondroitin, Vitamin C
Leiner Health Products, Inc.
www.yourlifevitamins.com
800-533-8482

ZonePerfect

Fish oils: Omega-3 fatty acids (EPA & DHA)
ZonePerfect Nutrition Co.
www.zoneperfect.com
978-232-9400

Online resources

ConsumerLab.com

This web site offers online subscribers access to product reviews including those in this book as well as new reviews and updates. It also provides recent and archived recalls and warnings and a comprehensive encyclopedia of natural products and drug interactions. Readers will find free general information as well as subscription-only content. www.consumerlab.com

Government resources

THE SPECIAL NUTRITIONALS ADVERSE EVENT MONITORING SYSTEM

Here, readers can find adverse event (illness or injury) reports associated with use of a special nutritional product: dietary supplements, infant formulas, and medical foods. The information comes from the U.S. Food and Drug Administration's (FDA's) MedWatch program; the FDA's field offices; other federal, state, and local public health agencies; and letters and phone calls from consumers and health professionals. Reporting is voluntary and the information is as reported by the consumer or health care professional. Unfortunately, online information hasn't been updated since October 1998.
http://vm.cfsan.fda.gov/~dms/aems.html

FDA ENFORCEMENT REPORT INDEX

This web site is published weekly by the FDA. It contains information on actions taken in connection with agency regulatory activities.
http://www.fda.gov/opacom/Enforce.html

MEDWATCH: REPORTING ADVERSE EVENTS

MedWatch allows both health care professionals and consumers to report serious problems that they suspect are associated with drugs and medical devices. Reporting can be done online, by phone, or by submitting the MedWatch 3500 form by mail or fax.
http://www.fda.gov/medwatch/how.htm

INDEX

t refers to a table

Index

t refers to a table

t refers to a table

t refers to a table

t refers to a table

t refers to a table

t refers to a table

t refers to a table

t refers to a table

t refers to a table

Supplement, 79t

WXYZ

Walgreens Finest Gin-Zing
Concentrate, 129t

Walgreens Ginkgo Biloba
Standardized Extract, 125t

Walgreens Multiple Vitamins with
Iron One Daily for Adults and
Children, Dietary Supplement,
43

Walgreens Pharmaceutical Grade
Calcium Magnesium, 87t

Walgreens Saw Palmetto
Standardized Extract, 148t

Walgreens Vitamin C with Rise Hips,
74t

Whole Foods Chelated iron, 93t

Windmill Natural Rose Hips with
Vitamin C, 74t

Windmill Vitamin E, 79t

Wormwood, hazards of, 26

Yerba Prima St. John's Wort Extra
Strength Herbal Supplement,
161t

Yohimbe, hazards of, 26

Your Life Coenzyme Q10 30 mg
Supplement, 102t

Your Life Ginkgo Biloba
Standardized Herbal Extract,
125t

Your Life Natural Oyster Shell
Calcium with Vitamin D, 87t

Your Life Natural Vitamin C, 74t

Zinc, 53

in multis, problems with, 35

ZonePerfect Omega 3 Molecular
Distilled Fish Oil and Vitamin E
Supplement, 118t